The Kentucky Bicentennial Bookshelf
Sponsored by

KENTUCKY HISTORICAL EVENTS CELEBRATION COMMISSION

KENTUCKY FEDERATION OF WOMEN'S CLUBS

and Contributing Sponsors

AMERICAN FEDERAL SAVINGS & LOAN ASSOCIATION

ARMCO STEEL CORPORATION, ASHLAND WORKS

A. ARNOLD & SON TRANSFER & STORAGE CO., INC. / ASHLAND OIL, INC.

BAILEY MINING COMPANY, BYPRO, KENTUCKY / BEGLEY DRUG COMPANY

J. WINSTON COLEMAN, JR. / CONVENIENT INDUSTRIES OF AMERICA, INC.

IN MEMORY OF MR. AND MRS. J. SHERMAN COOPER BY THEIR CHILDREN

CORNING GLASS WORKS FOUNDATION / MRS. CLORA CORRELL

THE COURIER-JOURNAL AND THE LOUISVILLE TIMES

COVINGTON TRUST & BANKING COMPANY

MR. AND MRS. GEORGE P. CROUNSE / GEORGE E. EVANS, JR.

FARMERS BANK & CAPITAL TRUST COMPANY / FISHER-PRICE TOYS, MURRAY

MARY PAULINE FOX, M.D., IN HONOR OF CHLOE GIFFORD

MARY A. HALL, M.D., IN HONOR OF PAT LEE,

JANICE HALL & MARY ANN FAULKNER

OSCAR HORNSBY INC. / OFFICE PRODUCTS DIVISION IBM CORPORATION

JERRY'S RESTAURANTS / ROBERT B. JEWELL

LEE S. JONES / KENTUCKIANA GIRL SCOUT COUNCIL

KENTUCKY BANKERS ASSOCIATION / KENTUCKY COAL ASSOCIATION, INC.

THE KENTUCKY JOCKEY CLUB, INC. / THE LEXINGTON WOMAN'S CLUB

LINCOLN INCOME LIFE INSURANCE COMPANY

LORILLARD A DIVISION OF LOEW'S THEATRES, INC.

METROPOLITAN WOMAN'S CLUB OF LEXINGTON / BETTY HAGGIN MOLLOY

MUTUAL FEDERAL SAVINGS & LOAN ASSOCIATION

NATIONAL INDUSTRIES, INC. / RAND MCNALLY & COMPANY

PHILIP MORRIS, INCORPORATED / MRS. VICTOR SAMS

SHELL OIL COMPANY, LOUISVILLE

SOUTH CENTRAL BELL TELEPHONE COMPANY

SOUTHERN BELLE DAIRY CO. INC.

STANDARD OIL COMPANY (KENTUCKY)

STANDARD PRINTING CO., H. M. KESSLER, PRESIDENT

STATE BANK & TRUST COMPANY, RICHMOND

THOMAS INDUSTRIES INC. / TIP TOP COAL CO., INC.

MARY L. WISS, M.D. / YOUNGER WOMAN'S CLUB OF ST. MATTHEWS

Medicine in Kentucky

JOHN H. ELLIS

THE UNIVERSITY PRESS OF KENTUCKY

For Wanda

Research for The Kentucky Bicentennial Bookshelf
is assisted by a grant from the
National Endowment for the Humanities.
Views expressed in the Bookshelf do not
necessarily represent those of the Endowment.

ISBN: 0–8131–0232–4

Library of Congress Catalog Card Number: 76-51156

A statewide cooperative scholarly publishing agency
serving Berea College, Centre College of Kentucky,
Eastern Kentucky University, The Filson Club,
Georgetown College, Kentucky Historical Society,
Kentucky State University, Morehead State University,
Murray State University, Northern Kentucky University,
Transylvania University, University of Kentucky,
University of Louisville, and Western Kentucky University.

Editorial and Sales Offices: Lexington, Kentucky 40506

Contents

Preface

THE PURPOSE OF this book is to present a brief history of Kentucky medicine from early times to the present. Such a purpose imposes severe limitations, and I have confined the account mostly to the development of professional institutions. It is both surprising and unfortunate that so little has been done on the subject, for the sources are exceedingly rich. Some indication of Kentucky's treasures for medical history is offered in the Bibliographical Note.

It is common knowledge that the annals of Kentucky history are filled with names of giants in American medicine: Daniel Drake, Ephraim McDowell, Benjamin W. Dudley, Samuel D. Gross, and others. However, following the example of the compilers of an earlier work, I have made no attempt "to overshadow the useful activities of the many with the brilliant genius of a few." Neither has any distinction been made between Kentucky's native medical sons and her adopted ones. In May 1879 at Danville, while presenting the door-knocker from Ephraim McDowell's home to Samuel D. Gross, a native of Pennsylvania then residing in Philadelphia, Dr. Richard O. Cowling of Louisville spoke for the Commonwealth: "She will ever claim you as her son, and will look with jealous eye upon those who would wean you from her dear affection. And, as this emblem which is now given to you hangs no longer in a Kentucky doorway, by this token you shall know that all Kentucky doorways are open at your approach."

Many people have been very helpful to me in this undertaking, and it is a pleasure to acknowledge their kind, patient assistance. They are, in Louisville, Mr. Martin F. Schmidt, Mrs. Mettie Watson, and Mr. James R. Bentley, of the Filson

Club; Mrs. Joan Titley Adams and her staff, especially Mrs. Mary H. Stahl, of the Kornhauser Health Sciences Library, and Mr. Frank W. Shook, Jr., assistant director of Biomedical Educational Resources, Health Sciences Center, University of Louisville; in Frankfort, Mrs. Anne McDonnell of the Kentucky State Historical Society; in Lexington, Miss Roemol Henry, librarian, Frances Carrick Thomas Library, Transylvania University; Dr. Jacqueline Bull, now retired but formerly head, Special Collections, Margaret I. King Library, University of Kentucky; Mr. Scott Donovan and Miss Doris Scripture, Office of Continuing Education, and Miss Deborah Rankin, Office of Public Information, Albert B. Chandler Medical Center, University of Kentucky; and, in Bethesda, Maryland, Mrs. Dorothy Hanks, History of Medicine Division, National Library of Medicine. I also appreciate the cooperation of Mr. Thomas P. Summers, executive director of the Kentucky Lung Association; Mr. Robert G. Cox, executive director of the Kentucky Medical Association; and William P. McElwain, M.D., commissioner of Health Services, Kentucky State Department for Human Resources.

Three generous friends shared their own research and thoughts with me: Professor Martin Kaufman of Westfield, Massachusetts, on medical education in the United States; Professor James G. Burrow of Abilene, Texas, on the organizational work of Dr. Joseph N. McCormack for the American Medical Association during the early years of the twentieth century; and Eugene H. Conner, M.D., of Louisville, Kentucky, on various aspects of medicine in Kentucky. Dr. Conner also read this essay in manuscript and made many valuable suggestions. One is fortunate to have such friends.

Finally, I want to thank Mrs. Theresa Racosky, who typed the manuscript, and to express grateful appreciation for financial assistance from the Office of Research, Lehigh University, and from the Penrose Fund of the American Philosophical Society.

1

THE FRONTIER BACKGROUND

THE BEGINNINGS OF Kentucky medicine are to be found in the movement of colonial culture to the western frontier during the last quarter of the eighteenth century. This culture embraced traditions regarding disease, self-treatment, the physician, and medical practice, although evidences of an American medical profession as such, influenced to any appreciable extent by currents in European medical thought, did not appear until about the time of the Revolution. By way of setting the stage for later developments, a brief survey of the cultural background and its early movement to Kentucky is in order.

Among many prospects early settlers thought they perceived in the new land was an Eden of health. From the first settlement of Virginia through the eighteenth century, white immigrants and black slaves of differing genetic and immunologic backgrounds brought various diseases to the colonies. The fluxes, fevers, and pleurisies of "seasoning"—a continuous process of biosocial adaptation—were early names for dysentery and other enteric disorders, malaria, and respiratory diseases. These became endemic and were the principal causes of sickness and mortality. Generally epidemics were mitigated by the dispersion of population in regions having few principal cities. Yet even in remote rural areas smallpox, diphtheria, scarlet fever, measles, whooping cough, and mumps were infectious diseases not to be viewed lightly.

The mirage of health continued to recede with the frontier as Kentucky settlers transported their diseases to the new setting. Aside from economic and social factors, geological and topographical characteristics were also significant in establishing disease patterns. For example, proximity of limestone strata to water sources favored the spread of dysentery and other enteric maladies, and the high mineral content of spring waters caused calculous disease of the genitourinary tract.

According to the famous physician Daniel Drake, "From the earliest period of its settlement the whole plateau, from the Falls to Salt River, has been infested with autumnal fevers, intermittent and remittent, simple and malignant."[1] In what came to be called the "poor south" and in the northcentral hill country, typhoid was an especially frequent and often fatal visitor. In backwoods areas, where cows fed on herbage including the white snakeroot, settlers contracted that deadly and perhaps most terrifying of all pioneer diseases, milk sickness. Smallpox came with the westward movement, prevailing as an epidemic in Lexington during the winter of 1793/1794.

In remote and sparsely settled areas of the colonies, and later on the Kentucky frontier, home treatment and self-medication in times of illness were the rule. During pioneer days in Hardin County, wrote an early resident, "the women were the doctors."[2] The complete housewives of that time delivered babies, bound up wounds, and treated fevers with traditional recipes—teas made from local herbs, various Indian remedies, and sometimes a few proprietary or patent medicines. Though maligned by medical contemporaries, the ministrations of early "doctresses" may have been as skillful and efficacious as those of most physicians following established practices in treatment.

The colonial physician descended from a line of ships' surgeons, and he resembled the rural English surgeon-apothecary, who was a general practitioner. A few sons of wealthy parents went abroad for formal medical education in

2

the European centers of Leyden, London, and Edinburgh. But it is estimated that at the time of the Revolution only about 400 of approximately 3,500 colonial practitioners held the M.D. degree. The overwhelming majority were trained by apprenticeship, usually for four years or more though the period became shorter in time, to a physician who most often was himself apprentice-trained. Under this arrangement the preceptor provided his student with practical experience and such theoretical knowledge as he possessed, and in return the student assisted his preceptor in practice, performed various chores, and paid him a fee. Whether the student was well or ill trained depended on the ability and conscientiousness of his preceptor.

Apprenticeship, then, was the traditional mode of medical education that carried over to the Kentucky frontier. In 1788 the well-known surveyor, town builder, and schoolmaster, John Filson, drew up an agreement between himself and "Doctr. John Toms Slater," who had recently arrived at Lexington station. Its terms required Slater to establish an apothecary shop, procure medicines, and house "a student in Physic, surgery &C to said Doctor Slater, he Covenanting and engageing to instruct said Filson to the extent of his knowledge and ability in all the knowledge, & Mistery, of the theory and practice of Physic, Surgery, and midwifery, also the full use of his books on Physic, Surgery, &C during Said term of two years: for which, and on account thereof, Said Filson shall pay said Doctor Slater the sum of twenty pounds, as a fee."[3] Though the agreement was never consummated, it is nonetheless typical of the character of early medical training.

Since university-educated English physicians rarely emigrated to the colonies and but few young men went to Europe for medical education, colonial medical thought and practice were dominated by traditions dating back to the second-century Greek physician Galen. In these traditions distinction was made between different states or conditions observed in sick persons but not between diseases as such. The morbid condition of illness was explained by theories concerning an imbalance of body humors or fluids (humoralism) or by the alternative concept of tense and relaxed states in the body's solid parts (solidism). Galenic humoral doctrine prevailed, however, and colonial practitioners employed therapies to alter body conditions such as fevers or fluxes rather than to treat particular diseases.

Depending on whether the humors (black bile, yellow bile, blood, and phlegm) were thought to be disordered by impurities or by imbalance through excess or deficiency, the physician treated illness by depletion (sweating, purging, and bleeding) or by restoring the body with diet and stimulant tonics. Standard remedies acquired from tradition and practical experience included known vegetable and mineral drugs as well as some Indian preparations. While this materia medica was small by present standards, most physicians practiced an aggressive polypharmacy even then.

Surgery performed by colonial doctors was limited mostly to amputations, treatment of superficial wounds and growths, and the setting of fractures and dislocations. A few men were skilled in the ancient practice of cutting for stone (removal of calculous stones from the urinary bladder), but the risk of infection from penetration of the body's interior cavities was great. Thus, the principal elements of medical practice in colonial times and on the Kentucky frontier were traditional therapy and limited surgery.

On the business side physicians were compensated by fee-for-service both in cash and in labor, livestock, or produce. However, even when doctors' bills were paid promptly and in full, the average income from medical practice was low, a situation due primarily to a surplus of practitioners who derived only part of their incomes from "doctoring." Medical practice was not uncommonly combined with storekeeping, farming, preaching, and other lines of endeavor. This was the case with the Virginia physician-surveyor, Dr. Thomas Walker, who explored areas of Kentucky during the 1750s.

By the time of the Revolution there were evidences of emerging medical institutions and the beginnings of a profession. These evidences included the formation of colonial, and later state, medical societies; the beginnings of medical publications; and the establishment of formal medical education at the University of Pennsylvania. These developments show a certain maturing of colonial culture through the influence of currents in European medical thought.

Lacking the restraints imposed on European physicians by their professional guilds, colonial doctors often competed fiercely in practice and were generally regarded as a contentious, quarrelsome lot. Beginning with New Jersey in 1766, the first provincial medical societies sought to distinguish between qualified and unqualified practitioners through apprenticeship requirements and through examination and licensing procedures. Physicians who held the M.D. degree were usually exempt from examination, and in most places the degree itself was a license to practice. The early societies also sought to promote harmony and accord among the qualified practitioners by personal association and by voluntary control of professional competition through adherence to uniform fee schedules. These efforts were fairly successful in the older states. One attraction of the Kentucky frontier was the absence of such restraints.

Another significant aspect of professional development was accessibility to and the increase of medical publications. By the 1750s a number of English medical journals were available to colonial physicians both as readers and as contributors. Following the Revolution similar publications were established in the United States. Among the more important early periodicals was the Philadelphia *Eclectic Repertory*, a journal destined in later years to publish a landmark report of three successful ovariotomies performed by a Danville, Kentucky, surgeon named Ephraim McDowell. Like the medical societies, the publications reflected professional self-consciousness of a rising level of medical education.

Despite relative isolation from trends in European scientific and medical thought during the seventeenth and early eighteenth centuries, colonial society remained aware of the M.D. degree's prestige. An increasing flow of students going abroad for medical education after 1740 leavened colonial medicine with the ideas of Thomas Sydenham, the seventeenth-century

"English Hippocrates," who rejected traditional humoral doctrine and postulated an ontological concept of disease as a specific entity existing apart from man. The contributions of Hermann Boerhaave, the great Dutch teacher-clinician at Leyden, also had significant impact. But the dominant influence on late colonial medical thought was the University of Edinburgh and the teaching of William Cullen. Like Sydenham, Cullen rejected humoral theory, but unlike his predecessor he revived traditional solidist doctrine by assuming that the basic factor in health and disease was a "nervous force." The disordered state of this force was "debility," a condition curable by therapy that induced relaxation. In 1765 the Edinburgh University pattern and Cullen's teaching were transported to Pennsylvania when John Morgan, an Edinburgh graduate, established the first American medical school, as an adjunct to the College of Philadelphia.

By requiring preliminary education for admission to what came to be known as the Medical Department of the University of Pennsylvania, Morgan intended to elevate the social and professional standing of the physician. His overall plan for the school was almost immediately successful, and within a few years he assembled a full medical faculty. This faculty included Benjamin Rush, famous as a patriot and signer of the Declaration of Independence, who was also a student of Cullen and an Edinburgh graduate. Rush combined Cullen's doctrines with theories of direct and indirect debility advanced by his fellow student John Brown and concluded that there was but one disease state, "morbid excitement," which he attributed to irregular action of the arterial system. The appropriate treatment, according to Rush, was a vigorous depletive therapy of puking, purging, and bleeding. The influence upon Kentucky medicine of the University of Pennsylvania and of this eminent and forceful teacher was both profound and of long duration.

There were only a few medical practitioners in Kentucky before 1800. The first is believed to have been Dr. George Hartt, who emigrated from Maryland to Harrod's station in

1775, moved near Louisville a few years later, and finally settled in Bardstown. After the Revolution colonial army officers, including surgeons and surgeons-mates, received sizable Kentucky land warrants as bounties for military service. Dr. Alexander Skinner, who is reported to have lived and practiced near the Louisville fort, served as a regimental surgeon in the Virginia Continental Line and received a land bounty of 6,000 acres. The first to establish permanent residence and practice in Lexington was Dr. Frederick Ridgley, a thirty-four-year-old veteran from Maryland, who came in 1790 and, except for service during Indian campaigns with General Anthony Wayne, remained until 1822.

The settlement of Kentucky proceeded rapidly between 1784, when John Filson reported the presence of 30,000 souls, and 1800, when the federal census of the fourteenth state showed a population of 220,955. During the interim years heavy inward migration down the Ohio River route and through the Cumberland Gap brought the families of Ephraim McDowell, Benjamin Winslow Dudley, and Samuel Brown from Virginia and that of Daniel Drake from New Jersey. These men became distinguished as physicians and teachers and played an important part in the growth of Kentucky medical institutions during the nineteenth century.

2

MEDICAL
EDUCATION

IN 1780 the Virginia General Assembly placed 8,000 acres of land confiscated from Loyalists under the control of trustees of a "seminary of learning" for the Kentucky district. Three years later the assembly formally named the institution Transylvania Seminary. For years there was constant controversy over the land and control of the school between rival interests having to do with Federalist-Republican politics and Presbyterian-Baptist denominational strife. Finally, in 1798, the Kentucky General Assembly commanded the peace, designated Lexington as the school's location, and renamed it Transylvania University. One of the first acts of new trustees in 1799 was to create the Medical Department by appointing Dr. Samuel Brown professor of chemistry, anatomy, and surgery, and Dr. Frederick Ridgley professor of materia medica, midwifery, and practice of physic. Thus began formal medical education west of the Alleghenies.

After years of vicissitudes during which no medical degrees were conferred, Transylvania assembled a full faculty in the Medical Department in November 1817 with a class of twenty students. This original faculty included Benjamin W. Dudley, M.D., who held two chairs, anatomy and surgery; James Overton, M.D., theory and practice of medicine; William H. Richardson, who would receive his M.D. degree in 1818, obstetrics and diseases of women and children; the Reverend James Blythe, D.D., chemistry; and Daniel Drake, M.D., who came from Cincinnati to accept the chair of materia medica. Aside from Dudley and Drake a contemporary considered the faculty to be "of moderate intellectual grade."[1] Unfortunately, there was trouble from the start.

By holding two chairs Dudley received two fees. He was on intimate terms with at least two trustees—Henry Clay and a former partner, Dr. James Fishback—and so he came to be "the reigning monarch of the Medical Department of Transylvania University."[2] Affecting the French manners of Napoleon's court, and bearing a diploma from London's Royal College of Surgeons, Dudley picked at Blythe and Richardson for lacking medical degrees until the latter challenged him to a duel. Drake, who had attended medical lectures at Pennsylvania with the two adversaries in 1805/1806, came to Lexington with a growing reputation in medicine, natural science, and belles-lettres, together with a sharp tongue and a taste for invective. When he resigned at the end of the session, Dudley accused him of reneging on a promise to stay two years. Drake replied mildly from Cincinnati on July 10, 1818, that Dudley was "a base and unprincipled villain." This quarrel had to wait until Dudley and Richardson fought a pistol duel, in which the latter was severely wounded but later recovered. Dudley then resumed his attack on Drake on September 25 with fresh accusations. Eleven days later Drake informed the reading public concerning his antagonist's character: "In my first interview, I perceived the ensigns of Paris foppery to have nearly obscured the slender stock of intellect on which they were engrafted;—while a closer inspection soon convinced me, that egotism, ignorance and sycophancy had formed within him an unholy alliance, and alternately guided the helm of his destinies."[3] This rejoinder silenced Dudley, but as a result of the whole affair Transylvania suspended medical instruction for the coming year.

The first session's uproar was played out against the backdrop of Lexington's declining fortunes. Development of steam navigation, completion of the National Road to Wheeling, and the beginnings of other internal improvements began to shift the center of economic gravity in Kentucky toward the river towns even before the Bluegrass center was jolted by the Panic of 1819. With manufactures and commerce falling off sharply, Lexington's leading men, some of whom were Transylvania trustees, seized upon the university, and especially its Medical Department, as a means to economic recovery.

Under a new president, the Reverend Horace Holley, a Bostonian, overseer of Harvard and a Unitarian clergyman, the medical faculty was reorganized for the 1819/1820 session. Charles Caldwell, M.D., came from Philadelphia as dean and professor of the institutes and materia medica. Samuel Brown, a former professor and presumably the first physician in the West to vaccinate against smallpox using cowpox matter, returned to the chair of theory and practice. Dudley resumed the two chairs of surgery and anatomy; Richardson, having received the M.D., was reappointed in obstetrics; and the Reverend Blythe again taught chemistry.

Believing he personally had brought Philadelphia medical learning to a place where the "soil had never undergone the slightest preparation," Caldwell later wrote: "I had under my direction, one of the most miserable Faculties of medicine . . . that the Caucasian portion of the human family can well furnish, or the human mind easily imagine." Aside from himself and Dudley, the professors were "little else than medical ciphers."[4] (This assertion included Brown, who had recommended Caldwell for the job!) But twenty years before, in 1799, Dr. Brown had begun Transylvania's medical library and acquired some philosophical apparatus with $500 authorized by the trustees for those purposes; it was in fact on prepared and even on seeded ground that Caldwell appealed successfully to the Kentucky legislature in 1820 for $10,000 to acquire additional books and apparatus.

Considering the personalities involved, Transylvania's medical faculty remained fairly stable until 1837. Brown quarreled with Dudley and left in 1825; Drake returned in 1823 to depart for the last time four years later. Dudley's brother-in-law, Charles Wilkins Short, M.D., came to the chair of materia medica and botany in 1825, and the following year John Esten Cooke, M.D., replaced Drake in theory and practice. When the Reverend Blythe resigned in 1831 to become president of Hanover College in Indiana, Caldwell secured the chair of chemistry for his former pupil, Lunsford P. Yandell, M.D., a young Tennessean.

The first lectures by a full faculty were given in rooms above a tavern on what is now Short Street. Dudley lectured and demonstrated in his office (still standing on the corner of Mill and Church streets), to which he added a spacious amphitheater to accommodate medical classes that grew from 37 in 1819/1820 to 281 for the 1825/1826 session. Some of Lexington's more prominent citizens, together with a few professors, built Medical Hall on the corner of Market and Church streets adjacent to Dudley's amphitheater in 1827. For use of the new building the faculty paid an annual fee equal to 6 percent of construction costs.

Lectures were given six days a week beginning the first Monday in November and ending early in March. Students paid fifteen dollars for each professor's ticket; five dollars for a matriculation and library ticket; five dollars for a dissection ticket; and, for graduation, a fee of twenty dollars. In addition to the "public" lectures, professors also conducted "private" classes which, though not mandatory, seem to have been well attended at fees of about fifty dollars per session. For graduation the male student was required to be twenty-one years old, of good moral character, to have studied under a preceptor for two years, to have attended two courses of lectures (the last one at Transylvania), and, finally, to have submitted an acceptable thesis bearing on some branch of medicine. Physicians showing evidence of reputable practice for four years might become candidates for the M.D. degree after completing one course of lectures.

The years of the Reverend Holley's administration at Transylvania, 1818–1827, were the Medical Department's golden age. Brown and Cooke expounded forcefully the doctrines of Benjamin Rush, and while one student considered the Reverend Blythe "too exclusive and taciturn," he also believed him to be "a firm and good teacher."[5] Caldwell, absorbed in personal vanity, was an elegant, eloquent lecturer, but a former pupil recalled that students "turned listlessly away from his polished discourses on Sympathy, Phrenology, the Vital Principle, and other kindred themes, and hurried off to the lectures on Materia Medica and Anatomy" given by Drake and Dudley.[6]

Surviving M.D. theses indicate that the faculty had a strong influence on students, but not a stifling one. Writing in 1822, Henry G. Doyle of Louisville reflected on Adam Smith's view of universities as "the dull repositories of exploded opinion" and concluded, "Happily however for the students of Transylvania University, no such aristocratical principles are cherished here." Doyle then proceeded to attack Caldwell's teaching of unfavorable prognosis in medical jurisprudence as "mean and illiberal." Another student, seeking to elucidate the cause, pathology, and treatment of hysteria in women, found conflict between the theoretical formulations of traditional authorities and his own observations of comparable symptoms in males, who had no uterus, and concluded that medical practice in this regard was "to say the least, in some measure, unhappy & pernicious."[7] While tolerant of well-reasoned dissent, the faculty did not countenance dishonesty. Following commencement in 1827 it was discovered that a student had copied the thesis of a former graduate. The faculty ordered him to return for a third course of lectures—and he did!

Medical student life was as colorful as the glittering culture of the "Athens of the West" and, like Lexington's economic foundations, was somewhat precarious. Students risked life and limb when attempting to "resurrect" bodies from the local Baptist cemetery; one later recalled a night visit to Nicholasville during which "we were pursued when making way to the horses hitched outside [the] fence, and one ball of several lodged in the subject on my back."[8] Lexington's cultural life and her belles offered more pleasant diversion, and in 1821 a concerned uncle, Dr. Samuel Brown, urged his nephew Orlando not to neglect "true science." The uncle was obviously relieved the next year when his nephew gave up medicine for politics, a field "where your merits, whatever they may be, must meet with a just reward."[9]

By the early 1830s Louisville and Cincinnati were growing rapidly, but Lexington's population was only slightly more than 5,000 and a pall of what one observer termed "decreptitude [sic] and decline" hung over the city.[10] Despite the Reverend Holley's imaginative leadership, controversy and strife erupted in 1823, when he began to be attacked by a strange coalition of neo-Federalist Presbyterians and Baptists, backed by Governor Joseph Desha. Holley finally resigned in 1827, yet in the interim, according to Constantine Samuel Rafinesque, Transylvania's colorful and eccentric professor of botany and natural history, the charged atmosphere made for "little subordination among the students." In the Medical Department, where rivalry and factionalism were constant, "the Professors were far from being friendly with each other."[11] The university academic building burned in 1829; the Louisville-Portland canal was completed in 1831; Clay's Maysville road scheme went down under President Andrew Jackson's veto in 1832; and the next year Lexington was struck by a terrifying cholera epidemic. In 1836, with the clouds of a national depression on the horizon, word got around that the faculty planned to move the medical school to Louisville.

There may have been faculty who were dissatisfied with the difficulty of obtaining cadavers for dissection and with Transylvania's lack of a clinical teaching facility, but the overriding consideration was Lexington's economic decline. Apparently all the medical faculty were involved in the scheme initially, but facing the wrath of outraged citizens and trustees, Dudley and two ambitious young assistant professors, James M. Bush and Robert Peter, denounced Caldwell, Yandell, and Cooke as conspirators. Accusations of faithlessness, base treachery, cupidity, cowardice, and avarice were hurled at respective "hireling scribblers" and "imbecile beasts of prey" in the ensuing verbal melee. The trustees summarily dismissed Caldwell as the chief instigator and then on March 24, 1837, temporarily dissolved the entire faculty. That fall Caldwell, Yandell, and Cooke taught during the opening session of the Louisville Medical Institute. According to Dr. Robert Peter, the new professor of chemistry at Transylvania, all the trouble had come about from a lack of "harmony, necessary to efficient cooperation."[12]

Chartered in 1833, the Louisville Medical Institute began its first session in November 1837, with Caldwell in institutes and clinical practice, Yandell in materia medica, and Cooke in theory and practice, joining Jedediah Cobb, M.D., in anatomy, Joshua B. Flint, M.D., in surgery, and Henry Miller, M.D., in obstetrics and diseases of women and children. Charles W. Short came to the chair of materia medica, Yandell moving to chemistry, when the school's new Greek Revival building, providing better facilities for instruction and for the library, was completed in 1838. Also, the new school offered something the Lexington institution did not. Although Transylvania's medical faculty had served as attending physicians at the Kentucky Eastern Lunatic Asylum since its opening in 1824, there was no clinical instruction for students. Clinical teaching in the Louisville Marine Hospital, founded twenty years before, began with the new school. According to a second-year student who walked its wards "no symptom, however trivial, obscure, or mysterious, could pass unnoticed."[13]

Fees and graduation requirements were the same as those at Transylvania. In this respect both schools compared with other medical colleges of the time. A Nelson County physician gave his son the large sum of $410 in 1841 to attend medical lectures in New York, but most Kentucky families preferred the lower cost of a western medical education. However, the Louisville student, especially one attending his first course, always needed some new textbook requiring money from home. Wherewithal in hand, he then devoted himself to anatomical examination of oysters and to dissections of pigs' feet and grouse. His inductive studies of alcohol chemistry preceded loud recitations on city streets during the early morning hours, which brought him escort to the watchhouse where he and other students named John Smith soon stood before the mayor's court. But the second-course student was a man transformed. His serious face could be seen on the front bench as he listened intently, taking copious notes, and, bedazzled by professorial erudition, asking for detailed explanations of the lecturer's favorite theory. Just before graduation examinations he made it a point to acquire the odor of the dissecting room in order to impress the professors, hoping thereby to obtain the M.D. degree. The diploma in hand, wrote one student, was "a free permit to kill whom I pleased without the fear of the law."[14]

Unfortunately, the same sort of personal and factional enmities that split Transylvania continued unabated in Louisville. Daniel Drake recalled boyhood cornhusking bees as the source of his learning that "competition is the mother of cheating, falsehood and broils" and remembered that candidates for the job of schoolhouse waterboy "were as numerous and as vigilant as the candidates for professorships in our medical schools." From the outset the Louisville Medical Institute, renamed the Medical Department of the University of Louisville in 1846, came under bitter attack by the city's physicians, and the school's faculty responded in kind. Drake came back to the state from Cincinnati in 1839 to join such personalities as Caldwell and Yandell, known respectively to be vain and aggressive, and Henry Miller, who "was fond of disputation." The next year Caldwell conspired to undermine Flint's position in surgery, and when Flint resigned Drake obtained the post for his friend, Samuel D. Gross. Amid the ruckus created by Flint's partisans and foes, Gross recalled, "my reception by the medical profession of Louisville was anything but cordial."[15] Conditions were such that Drake and Cobb threatened to resign in 1843, and although Cooke's retirement under pressure in 1844 hardly stirred the waters, Caldwell's similar fate five years later produced a vindictive exchange of parting blasts.

From its inception the Louisville Medical Institute was decidedly influenced by the early-nineteenth-century school of French clinical pathology whose leading members—Bichat, Corvisart, Laennec, and Louis, to mention a few—sought to establish a precise correlation between bedside clinical findings and organic lesions revealed by autopsy. The concept of specific disease entities advanced by their quantitative method in pathology eventually supplanted the earlier doctrines of Cullen and Rush. The retirements of Cooke and Caldwell mark the transition in medical thought. Elisha Bartlett, a pupil of Louis and the outstanding American exponent of French contributions, taught at both Transylvania and the Louisville school during the 1840s, a time of changing fortunes for the two institutions.

In a letter of May 12, 1838, urging a former colleague to join the faculty in Louisville and predicting a bright future for the new school, Yandell expressed his belief that "Dr. Dudley's fame may enable Transylvania to vie with the Institute for a year or two; but it cannot withstand everything." When the Louisville school built a new clinical amphitheater next to the Marine Hospital in 1840, Transylvania erected a new Greek Revival Medical Hall the same year. But Yandell's prophecy was correct. Transylvania barely held its own until 1844, when Dudley finally surrendered the chair of anatomy to his longtime assistant, James M. Bush. Enrollment dropped from 254 in 1840/1841 to 169 in 1847/1848, while Louisville's classes rose from 205 to 406. In 1850 Dudley relinquished the chair of surgery at Transylvania and retired fully to what Gross later called "a species of gradually increasing imbecility."[16] That year the Lexington school had but 92 medical students.

At this juncture Joshua B. Flint, who formerly taught surgery in the Louisville Medical Institute, together with Henry M. Bullitt, professor of materia medica at Transylvania, contrived a plan to start a second medical school in Louisville in hopes of saving the one in Lexington. Arrangements were made to use the charter of a school at La Grange (Funk Seminary renamed Masonic University) to establish the Kentucky School of Medicine. Other than Flint, the entire faculty for the first three sessions beginning in the fall of 1850 was Transylvania's. Meanwhile, Transylvania shifted to a spring session for which the faculty—and, it was hoped, their Louisville students—returned to Lexington. This development made it possible for students to obtain the M.D. degree in less than one calendar year and thus marked the beginning of a decline in educational standards. Both schools used Benjamin W. Dudley's name as emeritus professor of surgery and cut fees sharply as inducements, but the attempt to save Transylvania proved unsuccessful. In 1854 Professors James M. Bush, Ethelbert L. Dudley, Robert Peter, Thomas D. Mitchell, and Llewellyn Powell resigned their chairs in the Kentucky School of Medicine, the first three returning to Transylvania to conduct fall and spring sessions until 1856. On February 7, 1859, the Lexington school held its last commencement, for six students in a class of twenty-three. Just below that entry in the matriculation record book Dr. Robert Peter wrote: "And so ended the first cycle of the Medical Department of Transylvania University."[17]

During the early 1840s Transylvania and the Louisville Medical Institute ranked just behind the University of Pennsylvania as the largest medical schools in the country. The flush times passed, however, and by the late 1850s the University of Louisville Medical Department and the Kentucky School of Medicine competed desperately for students. Partisans of the former attacked the latter's charter; yet after the Transylvanians departed permanently, Dr. Bullitt and the other faculty members at KSM barely managed to hang on. The war years were particularly difficult for this school, and in 1866 one remaining trustee—who happened to be Bullitt's brother-in-law—arranged for consolidation of the two Louisville schools on condition of a professorship for his relative by marriage. The merger was brief, however, for when most of the former KSM faculty were sacked at the end of the 1866/1867 session "that which stalks in darkness and steps its coward tread at midnight was revealed." The trustee's act had been illegal and shortly the victims of "low trickery" and "shameless rodomontade" revived the KSM.[18] Two years later, in 1869, some younger physicians who had been military surgeons, including the fiery one-armed Confederate veteran from Virginia, Edwin S. Gaillard, organized the Louisville

17

Medical College. That fall UL cut its fees from $120 to $50, a portent of the bitter competition and controversy that lay ahead.

Between 1870 and 1900, an era often referred to as "the age of enterprise," the main arena of Kentucky medical enterprise was Louisville and its medical schools. Rancor between medical professors and the community's practitioners on the one hand and conflict between schools on the other were nothing new. But after the Civil War, owing mainly to an unstable national currency and severe fluctuations in the economy, competitive rivalries became more intense. Physicians who depended exclusively on medical practice for a livelihood began to see clearly that their interests conflicted with those of the professors who derived a substantial portion of their incomes from student fees while producing new competitors in the medical marketplace. During the state medical society's meeting at Bowling Green in 1870 one Louisville doctor offered a resolution endorsing recent American Medical Association recommendations for raising standards in medical education. An angry debate ensued between practitioners and professors, but the resolution passed by a vote of 18 to 11.

Meanwhile, the schools resorted to devious competitive methods and practices that lowered educational standards even further. The requirement of a thesis had been long since abandoned when the long tradition of apprenticeship began to be discarded in the commercial competition for student fees. Its existence already precarious and prospects doubtful, KSM followed UL's lead by cutting total fees, including thirty dollars for graduation, to ninety-five dollars for the 1870/1871 session. The new Louisville Medical College immediately attacked the "cheap fee schools" while establishing "beneficiary" scholarships (which virtually every student received) as a front for comparable fee reductions. UL professors exposed the clever scheme whereby LMC used congressmen, local officials, and civic leaders as drummers for students by giving them the deceitful impression that they had been selected to award a partial scholarship to some worthy lad. The result of all this for medical education may be inferred from the following episode:

In February 1872, Jacob Geiger from Missouri expressed his desire to come forward for graduation after attending one course of lectures at LMC. Being unable to show evidence of four years' previous reputable practice, and having allegedly told fellow students he had never practiced, his request was denied. Geiger then went over to UL where he was graduated the following month. Dean James M. Bodine claimed to have received satisfactory information from Geiger's preceptor, one Galen E. Bishop, and since the candidate met all other requirements, especially the financial ones, the M.D. degree "was dully [*sic*] conferred upon him."[19]

There was also a brief threat of renewed competition from Lexington. After the Civil War, Transylvania, Kentucky University in Harrodsburg, and the new Agricultural and Mechanical College were consolidated in Lexington under the name Kentucky University. Former Transylvania faculty including James M. Bush, Henry M. Skillman, and Robert Peter established a Medical Department in 1874, but it was discontinued when the university underwent reorganization four years later. Also in 1874, Central University at Richmond lent its name and charter to a fourth Louisville school, the Hospital College of Medicine. The UL faculty tried to head off this new competitor by proposing to operate it themselves as a spring session school using UL facilities, something like the Transylvania-KSM relation in the 1850s. But Central University rejected the proposal, and the Hospital College of Medicine, charging competitive fees, held its first session with a handful of students during 1874/1875.

Heightened competition and the battering effect of depression after 1873 drove KSM to the wall. Suspending its fall session in 1874, the school reorganized for a spring session in 1875 and moved in bag and baggage with LMC, Dr. Edwin S. Gaillard being dean of both. Fees remained the same; the graduate received a diploma from each school; no mention was made of the traditional requirement to be twenty-one years of age and of good moral character, although students were urged not to be absent frequently without special permission. Having failed earlier to make a similar arrangement with the

Hospital College of Medicine, UL righteously attacked the KSM-LMC "Lightning Express" as a disgrace to medical education. The KSM faculty subsequently defended the school's low standards by declaring that "the greatest blessings to medical science have been derived from those who entered the profession comparatively uneducated."[20] In June 1876, Dean Bodine of UL played a leading role in organizing the American Medical College Association at Philadelphia in an effort to use higher educational standards as a weapon in the local competitive struggle.

The KSM-LMC housekeeping arrangement lasted for another decade, but by 1879 the Louisville schools had become more responsive to demands for educational reform emanating from various quarters in the profession. That year all schools made graded courses (basic, intermediate, and advanced) available, and all but KSM claimed membership in the American Medical College Association. During the 1880s, moreover, reasonably harmonious relations among the schools resulted from a gentlemen's agreement to abandon fee competition and share the available pool of students equitably. And in 1888 medical education for Negroes began when, using the charter of State University founded in 1879 by the Colored Baptist General Association of Kentucky, a group of the city's black physicians including Dr. H. Fitzbutler and Dr. Rufus Conrad incorporated the Louisville National Medical College. Anticipating approval of the school's legal status, Dr. Fitzbutler and his associates introduced a three-year course in 1886 and graduated William T. Peyton of Louisville, the first black man to receive an M.D. degree in Kentucky, in 1889.

That same year the American Association of Medical Colleges reorganized under this new name, and two years later the National Conference of State Medical Examining and Licensing Boards adopted the three-year graded course as a standard in medical education. In 1893 under the new medical practice act the Kentucky State Board of Health was armed with tougher licensing authority. Hemmed in by the AAMC on the national level and by the State Board of Health on the local level, the Louisville schools had no choice but to capitulate. In its announcement for 1894/1895 UL reminded prospective students who had attended a course of lectures prior to September 1, 1893, of THE LAST OPPORTUNITY to obtain a degree by enrolling for one more course. The other schools followed suit, extending degree requirements to three years and embracing the modern age of medicine with courses in bacteriology, microscopy, and pathological histology. In 1898 UL introduced the four-year curriculum, and the following year it became a requirement.

By 1900 Louisville had seven medical schools, two of which were established in the 1890s. A group of homeopathic physicians, including Dr. C. P. Meredith and Dr. Allison Clokey, obtained a charter for the Southwestern Homeopathic Medical College in 1892. Among its distinguishing features was a female faculty member, Sarah J. Millsap, M.D., professor of hygiene and sanitary science, the first woman to teach in a Kentucky medical school. The Kentucky University Medical Department was born in 1898 when, following a schism in the Kentucky School of Medicine, departing faculty borrowed the charter of the state university in Lexington. Only nine of thirty-three matriculates graduated in 1899, explained the ensuing session's announcement apologetically, "because of a change from a three-year to a four-year course."[21]

At the turn of the century, leaders of Kentucky's medical profession regarded the state of medical education in the Commonwealth very much as Dr. John Morgan of Philadelphia had viewed it at the time of the Revolution. During the late 1880s and the 1890s there were in Louisville annually between 1,200 and 1,500 medical students, a motley, coarse "horde," according to one observer, which placed "white persons, colored persons, dogs, and medical students, in descending order of social acceptability."[22] The relative peace that had prevailed between institutions in the 1880s was broken when a city ordinance was adopted providing for equal footing of all schools (except the Louisville National Medical College) at City Hospital for purposes of clinical instruction. In 1895 the regular school faculties attempted to deny this right to students in the Southwestern Homeopathic Medical College.

After a bitter battle the regulars were forced to concede defeat when the hospital appointed two homeopathic graduates as interns. Morgan had believed that higher preparatory standards for medical education would elevate the economic and social status of the profession by conferring on the physician, as a Kentucky doctor put it more than a century later, "the refined and refining virtues of a *gentleman*."[23] Such virtues seemed lacking to Morgan in 1765 and, despite the developments of one hundred years in medical education, the profession's leadership in Kentucky believed they were lacking in 1900. During the early years of the twentieth century leading physicians would renew the quest for professional status through reconstruction of medical education.

3

DISEASE AND MEDICAL PRACTICE

ROMANTIC VERSIONS of the American frontier experience present a picture of hardy pioneers and robust, healthy farmers. But these nostalgic images of the past tend to conceal the real hardships of daily life, among which illness was one of the most common, during the settlement and growth of Kentucky in the nineteenth century. From the earliest times infectious diseases such as mumps, measles, whooping cough, scarlet fever, diphtheria, and, occasionally, smallpox, appeared on farms and in villages and towns. Some of them, especially diphtheria, took an awesome toll of life until well into the twentieth century. Pulmonary phthisis, or tuberculosis, and malaria became endemic at an early time and their respective standing as major killing and debilitating diseases has been lowered only in recent years.

Dysentery, or "bloody flux," also became endemic and, according to a Woodford County medical student writing in 1821, it hurried "to an untimely grave more than famine or the sword."[1] Diarrheal diseases prevailed extensively in most settlements from May through August, and recurrent waves of typhoid fever, particularly during dry summer seasons, swept over Kentucky with high fatality throughout the century. One Boyle County physician remembered that typhoid made 1843 "a prosperous year in the practice of medicine."[2] Influenza and pneumonia tended to prevail during fall and winter, the seasons most conducive to respiratory diseases, and these were also frequently fatal.

From time to time disease conditions exploded into epidemics. In 1822, "a sickly year over the West generally," Louisville inhabitants were stricken with a "bilious" affliction that may have been yellow fever.[3] Smallpox rarely presented a serious threat, but there were occasional outbreaks in towns and villages; one occurred in Lexington during 1849. In that same year Asiatic cholera struck Kentucky for the second time. The initial invasion in 1832 had been followed the next year by the spread of terror, death, and desolation from river towns to interior communities. Lexington was especially hard hit in June 1833, when cholera claimed nearly 150 victims in three days and a heroic vagrant called King Solomon shoveled day and night to bury the dead. The disease appeared in Bowling Green, Glasgow, and Greensburg in 1834 and decimated Russellville the following summer. After a fourteen-year abatement cholera returned between 1849 and 1854, attacking the river towns and, most severely, Lexington and Glasgow. Minor outbreaks occurred in 1866 on military posts near Louisville, Newport, and Bowling Green, but the overall effects were negligible. Then, in 1873, cholera ravaged Kentucky more severely than any other state. Five years later the great Mississippi Valley yellow fever epidemic of 1878 left a wake of suffering and death in the communities of Fulton, Hickman, and Bowling Green.

Among all diseases in a rural population, however, milk sickness inspired the greatest fear. Known from the times of earliest settlement, by the 1830s it prevailed conspicuously in Boone, Campbell, Breckinridge, Harrison, Daviess, and Ohio counties. The unknown cause was the white snakeroot (*Eupatorium rugosum*) on which cows foraged in the woods, producing what is now known to be tremetol poisoning. Suckling calves contracted it as did persons who consumed milk, butter, or flesh from stricken animals. Progressive symptoms in humans included lassitude, nausea, and vomiting followed by stomach pains and intense thirst. A swollen, white-coated tongue, subnormal temperature, and slow respiration were signs of oncoming prostration, coma, and death. One unfailing diagnostic indication was an unmistakable odor of the patient's breath and urine. Milk sickness was not only extremely likely to be fatal, but those who survived it seemed more susceptible to another attack and many never recovered normal health.

Medical students from the afflicted counties noticed that the disease was confined to wooded hill country farms and that cattle grazing on ground previously cultivated or woods recently burned over did not contract it. Where milk sickness or "the trembles" appeared, families abandoned their farms. In Boone and Campbell counties by 1824 many such farms remained unoccupied and were considered to have no value. In a report from Marshall County in western Kentucky, Dr. George W. Irvin of Benton noted in 1852 that "'milksickness' is so rife as to deter persons from purchasing property."[4] John Rowe, a Fayette County farmer, identified the cause of the disease as early as 1838, but not until 1917 did laboratory analysis prove he had been correct.

Dr. Benjamin W. Dudley observed in 1806 that treatment of female ills was "a very great part" of the Kentucky physician's practice. Frequent child-bearing and poor obstetrics were the principal factors and Dudley attributed much harm to "ignorant old women" midwives with their "whiskey stews" and "other nostrums." Another common female malady, hysteria, was said to be caused by diverse morbid phenomena acting upon the female economy and specifically the uterus. The disease was extremely complex, wrote a Transylvania medical student named John A. Ingles, who later became a successful Bourbon County practitioner, and "to enumerate all the symptoms, which have manifested themselves in different cases of hysteria, & which should therefore be considered hysterical, is more than I shall attempt."[5]

Dudley thought blacks were "most subject to those diseases which are the consequence of exposure to the weather, of an insufficiency in clothing, and of scanty and improper aliment," but he also believed they were prone to a distinct type of "consumption" not found in whites. Writing in 1832 a Tran-

25

sylvania medical student from Fayette County argued that "Negro Consumption" was neither so specific nor so distinct as physicians supposed. But blacks did in fact suffer heavily and disproportionately from respiratory diseases. Such ailments were "decidedly the most common" among them, noted a Louisville Medical Institute student during one of Daniel Drake's lectures in 1846, coming on "in the form of Pneumonia or Pleurisy." However, the Transylvania student also believed that much fatal illness among slaves resulted from "a too great dread of *Doctors Bills*" on the part of the owners and that neglect sent "to their long homes" many "who might have been saved by timely attention."[6]

Intemperate drinking, frequently a secondary cause of illness, and venereal disease were common health problems throughout the nineteenth century. When the temperance movement gained surprising strength in Kentucky during the 1840s, some doctors gave it their moral support. On May 12, 1847, Dr. Henry E. Guerrant of Sharpsburg, Bath County, and seventeen other men, received authority to create a local affiliate of the Grand Division of Kentucky, Sons of Temperance. Dr. Lemuel C. Porter, of Warren County, expressed pleasure in 1848 that the Sons of Temperance were "flourishing . . . and . . . exercising the most salutary influence over the habits of our citizens." Yet for all the good work, he thought, "it may be presumed that the task of total abstinence will be attended with much difficulty."[7]

Venereal disease was distinctive, according to a Lexington medical student, for its effect on "those organs *which every one prizes so highly*." Claiming gonorrhoea to be "one of the most common diseases[,] Yea! the most common in this beautiful and moral city," he went on to tell the story of a married patient who tried to evade his wife's wrath with the excuse of "having exchanged clothes with some one, or from the hole in a privy, or a strain." To illustrate venereal epidemiology the student offered the case of a local girl who was "considered a *fresh snap*, by many of the young bloods" and subsequently infected "upwards of 30" admirers.[8] As with intemperance, the cause of preventing venereal disease through total abstinence was attended with much difficulty.

Death rates based on various causes and diseases are difficult to establish for nineteenth-century Kentucky despite the enactment of a vital statistics law in 1851. It is reasonable to assume, however, that death rates prior to 1850 were very high compared to the present figure of 10 per 1,000, chiefly because of excessive infant mortality, and that these rates declined significantly between 1880 and 1900. In 1852 the Kentucky State Medical Society found mortality exceeding 2 percent, or 20 per 1,000, in the Bluegrass, north and northcentral Kentucky, and Livingston, McCracken, and Fulton counties in the far west. Little was known about the eastern mountain counties of the state where settlement was sparse and information not easily collected. Some idea of life expectancy at mid-century may be gained from a report of 61 deaths in Marshall County for the year ending June 1, 1850. The average age at death was 21.8 years.

The American tradition of self-dosage and home treatment was never stronger than during the early years of Kentucky settlement when there were relatively few trained physicians. Sometimes aided by domestic medical manuals, settlers purged themselves with calomel (mercurous chloride) and employed numerous homemade remedies. The measure of a large dose of calomel, according to a physician in a neighboring state, was one that "none but a Kentuckyan would give or take."[9] An "always successful" home recipe for treatment of dysentery called for two pounds of inner bark taken from the north side of a white oak tree. After boiling the bark with a gallon of water in an iron vessel until the liquid was reduced to a quart, the bark was removed, and to the remaining substance was added one quart of fresh milk and a lump of sugar as big as a duck egg. This mixture, in turn, was boiled down to a quart and, after cooling "a little," was ready for use. The dosage began with half a teacup followed by two tablespoons every two hours until distress in the lower tract and rectum abated. Practitioner and patient were advised to "then hold

27

on." If pains returned the regimen was repeated, but one course was said to be effective in most cases. Usually in a few days bleeding rectal ulcers would "slough off" and then the patient recovered. This recipe warned specifically against the use of calomel, "for if you do unlock the liver and let down bile upon the bleeding ulcers then you might as well speak for your coffin."[10] Nevertheless, calomel, home remedies, and patent medicines were the mainstays of home treatment throughout most of the nineteenth century.

Given the absence of legal restraints before 1874, medical practice was a wide-open enterprise. During the early years, especially, men combined "doctoring" with other lines of activity, notably preaching. Little is known of the Kentucky clergymen-physicians as a group, but they may have been fairly numerous for a brief period. At best they had regular training as did Dr. Caleb W. Cloud of Lexington, a Methodist preacher whose "ability and piety was only equalled by his eccentricity and independence."[11] At worst they may have resembled the Georgia preacher who, "like David, in an evil hour, fell into sin," shot the local sheriff, and escaped to Logan County near Russellville—then known as "Rogue's Harbor"—where he took up the practice of medicine.[12] Failure to distinguish between qualified and unqualified practitioners provided a fertile field for the charlatan. And soon the outright quack, who adhered to no system of pathology or therapeutics and usually promised miraculous cures, flourished in every part of the state.

By the 1830s four groups of practitioners, or sects, competed for medical practice in the United States. One group was composed of "regular," "orthodox," or "allopathic" physicians who practiced school medicine in the tradition of William Cullen and Benjamin Rush. A second group, "Indian doctors" or "herb doctors," was characterized by lack of formal education, opposition to regular therapeutics, and the use of botanic medicines. The third group, Thomsonian physicians, were much like the Indian doctors in that they lacked formal education and rejected regular therapeutics; they practiced a crude system of botanic therapy devised by a New Hampshire farmer named Samuel Thomson. The last group, known as homeopaths or homeopathic physicians, were formally educated in medicine but rejected orthodox pathology and therapeutics. They practiced a system of medicine devised by a German physician, Samuel Hahnemann, a system based on careful observation of symptoms, a principle of medicinal action known as the "law of similars," and the use of highly diluted uncompounded drugs.

Apart from the regular physicians, Indian doctors and Thomsonian practitioners were the most numerous. One well-known Thomsonian, Anthony Hunn, lived near Danville in Mercer County and acquired a considerable reputation in and around Danville, Harrodsburg, and Lancaster. Perhaps the most colorful Indian doctor was an adventurer named Richard Carter who settled near Versailles about 1815 and developed a remarkably extensive practice in Woodford, Jessamine, and surrounding counties before moving to Louisville in 1847. Neither Hunn nor Carter was a quack in any sense of the word. A present-day Kentucky medical historian, himself a physician, considers Carter to have been "a conscientious and useful member of the profession. . . . perhaps equal to the best of his professional brethren."[13] Thomsonian practice all but disappeared by the time of the Civil War, but a student of medical education in the United States in 1910 found the "yarb" doctor still entrenched in remote rural areas.

Though fewest in number, homeopathic physicians presented the most serious competitive threat to orthodox medical practice. Beginning in the 1840s regular physicians, including Dr. Henry Miller of the Louisville Medical Institute and Dr. Robert Peter of Transylvania, attacked homeopathy as a medical heresy, and medical journals termed it a "humbug." However, since this mode of practice was attractive mainly to a city-dwelling middle-class constituency, there were but few homeopathic physicians in Kentucky outside of Louisville and Lexington prior to the 1880s. By that time adherence to Hahnemann's rigorous doctrines and methods had deteriorated to the point that homeopathic and regular practice were hardly distinguishable. It is safe to say that while regulars and homeopaths engaged in bitter struggles in other parts of the nation throughout the nineteenth century, homeopathy was never a major force in Kentucky medicine.

With the establishment of medical education at Transylvania, the "heroic" therapeutics of Benjamin Rush became the distinguishing characteristic of regular medical practice. In the 1840s a young graduate of the Louisville Medical Institute caricatured the orthodox antiphlogistic regimen of purging, puking, and bleeding in most illnesses with a satire of his final examination in materia medica. Purgatives, he later wrote, were those "medicines whose action bears the same relation to that of emetics which the possums did to the hollow where the dog was waiting to catch them—they go the other way!" Calomel, "the four aces of medical murder," had been alluded to by Shakespeare in his injunction to "throw physic to the dogs" and yet again, though obscured by typographical error, where he wrote: "Be thou as pure as ice, as chaste as snow, thou shall not escape Calumel [calumny]." The effects of calomel upon the human system included "free use of coffins, spitboxes, mush-and-milk, and the invention of new oaths with which to curse the doctor!" Concerning emetics and their action, the former student described them as medicines a discreet man who had dined badly should not take. As for their action, it was like "that of money won at gambling—going back the way it came and taking a good deal more than it brought."[14] Another student subscribed to his professor's view that a single bleeding only aggravated a disease; more was better.

The students' caricature and testimonial alike describe accurately the standard therapies employed by regular physicians at the time. Dr. John Esten Cooke, professor of the theory and practice of medicine at both Transylvania and the Louisville Medical Institute for many years, is reported to have said: "If calomel did not salivate, and opium did not constipate, there is no telling what we could do in the practice of physic."[15] During Lexington's cholera epidemic in 1833, a time when doses of 60 to 80 grains were not uncommon, Cooke administered almost *one pound* of calomel to a patient in a single day. Doctors also used emetics liberally to evacuate the system and, when fever was present, they employed venesection, or bleeding, to reduce it by direct effect on the heart's action. Dr. Benjamin Dudley taught students to select the cephalic median vein in the arm and, using a sharp thumb lancet, to open it "till you see the blood rising."[16] The usual practice was to bleed until syncope, or fainting, occurred, but it was not uncommon for physicians to abstract as much as 50 ounces at a time. Cupping and counterirritant blisters were also employed to localize and counteract disease, measures which were both painful and likely to cause infection.

A classic example of mid-nineteenth-century Kentucky medical practice involved a young lady from Ohio who visited a Bowling Green family in 1852. When she became ill the family summoned a physician who diagnosed her case as influenza and began treatment with "bleeding cupping and mercurial." With the onset of chills over the next few days he administered quinine, more calomel, and ipecac, and repeated venesection and cupping along with blisters. On the thirteenth day of illness, according to the doctor's notes, the patient "was attacked with something resembling hysteria." During the next week her condition deteriorated under continued treatment and on the twenty-first day she died. "She was 20 years of age [and] of delicate constitution," wrote her physician. "She was amiable and beautiful[,] beloved by all who knew her and as much lamented in her death as the most favored in our land particularly by myself."[17]

Like this young woman, who was believed to be "inclined . . . to consumption," most tubercular patients were also treated with standard therapies. Skeptical of these methods Dr. John Croghan, an enterprising Louisville physician, bought Mammoth Cave in 1839 in the belief that its atmosphere would be beneficial to consumptives. Further encouraged by a colleague, Dr. William A. McDowell, who believed consumption could be cured, Croghan fitted up the cave in 1841 to receive patients. About fifteen persons participated in this novel experiment in the treatment of tuberculosis, but by the spring of 1843 most of them had died and the cave resort was an obvious failure. At the same time it was widely believed that mineral waters were efficacious in certain ailments where standard therapy had failed. Another enterprising physician, Dr. Christopher C. Graham, operated Harrodsburg Springs under his own name as a popular and financially successful health resort for over thirty years.

By midcentury the low repute of orthodox medicine was such, wrote one medical student, that there were "not wanting at the present day, men of intelligence and gravity, who seriously question whether the practice of physic does as much good as harm."[18] However, this situation was partly offset by some Kentuckians who made distinctive contributions to surgery. Walter Brashear, Richard Ferguson, and Charles McCreary gained eminence for both difficult and unprecedented operations. But the Nestor of early Kentucky surgeons was "the father of ovariotomy," Ephraim McDowell. The successful operation for ovarian tumor that McDowell performed Christmas Day, 1809, on Mrs. Jane Todd Crawford in Danville is a legend in the annals of Kentucky medicine. A talented operator, McDowell subsequently performed numerous ovariotomies among other surgical procedures throughout his distinguished career.

Another surgeon, Alban G. Smith, who was once McDowell's partner, pioneered in laminectomy, a procedure in spinal surgery. Joshua Taylor Bradford of Augusta succeeded to McDowell's eminence in ovariotomy, and Joshua Barker Flint, who taught in the Louisville Medical Institute, gained repute as a surgeon of exemplary competence. The most distinguished name in lithotomy, a procedure for removing stones from the urinary bladder, was that of Benjamin Winslow Dudley of the Transylvania Medical Department. Having studied firsthand the techniques of leading French and English surgeons, Dudley returned to Lexington in 1814 to win renown for his surgical feats. He is said to have performed 207 lithotomies with only 6 fatal results, a record which prompted Samuel D. Gross, himself a giant figure in surgery, to rank Dudley with Philip Syng Physick, John Collins Warren, and Valentine Mott as the greatest of American surgeons.

Dudley's habit of command learned from his father, a Revolutionary army officer turned Baptist preacher, applied to his patients also. He usually ignored their screams of pain, but if they struggled he is said to have warned: "Be still, Sir, or I'll send your soul to Hell in half a second." Like McDowell, Dudley practiced scrupulous cleanliness long before the era of antiseptic surgery. Both required that patients be carefully bathed before operations. In January 1847, just three months after the initial use of ether in Boston, Samuel B. Richardson was Kentucky's first surgeon to perform an operation using this form of anesthesia. Five years later an eminent physician reported that "in originality of conception and boldness of execution, Kentucky surgery may proudly challenge comparison with that of any of the older States in the Union."[19]

Even before the Civil War many of the therapeutic excesses of regular medicine were waning, and the century's closing decades brought the heyday of the country doctor and the appearance of specialization. The image of the rural practitioner of those years is frequently obscured by romance and myth, but often he was an excellent physician sincerely beloved by the people he served. Such a man, apparently, was Orrin D. Todd, a native of Shelby County who attended Jefferson Medical College in Philadelphia, graduating in 1865. After brief military service he started a practice in Eminence which won the community's confidence and spread into nearby counties. His striking personal appearance, affable manner, and skill as a physician and surgeon made his practice not only extensive but lucrative as well. When he died after a brief illness, the mayor of Eminence proclaimed all business closed the afternoon of Dr. Todd's funeral, May 5, 1896, and circuit court proceedings in New Castle were adjourned. Mourners estimated at 1,200 in number came from Louisville, Frankfort, Shelbyville, and outlying portions of Shelby County to pay their respects. Describing Dr. Todd as "one of God's noblemen," the local newspaper recounted how he had been "the happy, bright, sunny-natured physician at the bedside of the sick" and how he also "pressed the hands of the dying and made comfortable their last hours."[20]

A fairly good picture of rural practice in western Kentucky, if not of the man himself, may be seen in the account books of a Union County doctor. A native of Hancock County, Joseph E. Johnson attended the University of Notre Dame and graduated from the University of Louisville Medical Department in 1871. The next year he established a practice at Waverly in which he engaged actively until his death in 1916. From his account books it may be seen that Dr. Johnson treated white and black patients, recording his services and fees when he charged them. Usually, he charged one to two dollars for office visits and his fees in consultation ran from four to ten dollars. Tooth extractions were fifty cents and minor surgery, including fractures and dislocations, varied from eight to ten dollars.

Obstetrical work was the largest part of Johnson's busy practice, and for "visit to wife in labor" his charge from 1874 to 1898 was ten dollars. Some of his fees were paid in produce and work; the credit entries for "corn" are particularly numerous. In 1885, for example, John W. Roberts's debt was settled by "Pork $5.00"; James Hager obtained two dollars credit on account for work; treatment of Lewis McGuire's wife was settled by $4.46 cash and $7.54 credited to a calf; and Bryant Nichols paid his bill for $3.75 with a saddle. Altogether that year Dr. Johnson had accounts due of $1,385.96 for which he received $1,127.66.[21] This was probably a fairly good income by western Kentucky standards of that day.

The more prosperous country doctor practiced in an area of good farm land. Such was the case with Robert B. Pusey, M.D., of Elizabethtown in Hardin County. A native of Meade County, Pusey attended local schools and the academy at Brandenburg; he was graduated from Jefferson Medical College in Philadelphia in 1860. Soon afterward he married and began his practice in Elizabethtown. The couple had two sons, both of whom became distinguished physicians: William A. Pusey, M.D., an internationally famous dermatologist and his father's biographer, and Brown Pusey, M.D., a widely known Louisville ophthalmologist. From the older son's recollections of youth, and of his later experience assisting his father while a medical student, it is possible to know something about the practice of medicine in a moderately prosperous rural Kentucky district.

During the 1870s and 1880s Dr. Robert Pusey treated the same diseases his predecessors had confronted a half-century before: dysentery, typhoid fever, and respiratory infections, for the most part. A student of Samuel D. Gross at Jefferson, Pusey enjoyed surgery and did a great deal of it both in regular practice and through his work as a contract railroad surgeon. As with most country doctors, obstetrics made up a substantial portion of his work. Using chiefly the clinical thermometer, stethoscope, and various syringes and specula as instruments of physical diagnosis, Pusey also relied on his broad experience and keen sense-perception. Writing many years later the son concluded that his father has been a skillful diagnostician, but added: "I think, perhaps, he overworked the diagnosis of hysteria, as is so often done."[22]

In therapeutics Pusey's practice was comparable to that of most physicians in his day. The more common drugs he used included morphine, quinine, iodides, bromides, ergot, digitalis, aconite, and "barrels of syrup of rhubarb and potash with bismuth in acid dyspepsias."[23] During the late nineteenth century many of these elements of materia medica—morphine, quinine, and aconite, for example—came to be as much abused as calomel and ipecac at an earlier time. However Pusey, according to his son, did not give much medicine, preferring rather to rely on the body's natural healing powers. Believing in the efficacy of bed rest, he urged the value of clean bed linens and of a cheerful yet quiet and well-ventilated sickroom. A skillful surgeon, Pusey anesthetized his patients with chloroform, sometimes even to set fractures and dislocations, and, accepting the principle of bacteriology at least in surgery, he adopted a rough antiseptic technique using soap, water, and bichloride of mercury solution.

Like most country practitioners, Pusey kept no regular office hours since most of his time was spent in the buggy making calls. For these services the son believed his father's fees "were perhaps a little above the average."[24] Town visits and office calls were a dollar and up. Country trips involved regular fees plus a dollar for the first mile and fifty cents per additional mile. Consultations ran from five to twenty-five dollars; attending childbirth, ten dollars; minor surgical operations, five to twenty-five dollars; major operations (mainly amputations), twenty-five to one hundred dollars; and dislocations and fractures, ten to twenty-five dollars. From 1870 to 1886 Pusey's annual income averaged $5,200 in cash and other value, varying no more than $700 above or below that figure in any single year. By the standards of that day his practice was a lucrative one.

To his rural patients the country doctor was often the sole reliance in life's most desperate situations: a bad accident with axe or saw, a complicated labor, or a young child suddenly ill with fever. The doctor is sent for; family and neighbors wait around the porch watching the road. When he comes in sight the group's mood changes from anxiety to relief. The crisis has been met. Whatever the outcome, the doctor is there. Writing in Chicago in 1931, Dr. Pusey's son evaluated his father's rural Kentucky practice of an earlier day. There was a tendency, the son thought, to dismiss medicine before bacteriology as useless. Yet Robert Pusey's patients had never doubted his usefulness. Many times, perhaps, his ministrations brought no physical benefits, but he calmed fears, soothed griefs, cooled fevers, and relieved pains. Persons with lingering illnesses were made as comfortable as possible "and in such situations, to the great benefit of his patients, he did not add to their misery by trying to do more." The son concluded his father had been a good physician for whom patients felt gratitude and affection, adding, "Indeed the city doctor now, as a rule, has no such hold on the affection and confidence of his patients as doctors like Pusey had on theirs."[25]

The development of specialization was a cumulative result of the concept of specific disease entities, localized pathology and its concern for organs and organ systems, and technological development of instruments such as the ophthalmoscope, laryngoscope, and Roentgen ray for diagnostic purposes. Ophthalmology and surgery were early specialties whose practitioners had to overcome medical and social traditions which associated specialty with shady itinerant oculists and "cutters for stone" of a bygone day. Similarly, pioneers in the genitourinary field faced the moral opprobrium that long attached to venereal disease and stigmatized the specialist as a "clap doctor." But the rapid growth of cities after the Civil War as centers of transportation and industry, gathering together large populations and affording hospital facilities, provided the setting in which specialization flourished.

A prominent Kentucky doctor observed in 1881 that, in relation to the medical profession as a whole, "the specialists form the wings of the grand army, with which they move in harmonious co-operation, efficiency and success. . . . They are the aristocracy of medicine—their arena of action, our large cities."[26] Specialties developed most rapidly in Louisville, the center of medical education, and most of the early specialists were surgeons. Dr. Ap Morgan Vance, who had a special interest in orthopedics, was Kentucky's first physician to limit his practice to surgery. Other Louisville specialists in surgery whose careers spanned the late nineteenth and early twentieth centuries include David W. Yandell, James M. Holloway, A. M. Cartledge, William H. Wathen, William L. Rodman, Henry H. Grant, William O. Roberts, Lewis S. McMurtry, and Joseph M. Mathews, to name but a few.

On coming to Lexington in 1882 a young doctor from Missouri found local physicians so well established that it was difficult for a new man to get started. At that time the city's outstanding practitioners included Drs. John Whitney, David Barrow, Robert B. Waddy, Henry M. Skillman, and Joseph A. Stucky. The new arrival, Dr. Joseph W. Pryor, later recalled the welcome extended him by several colleagues, especially Dr. Stucky, who confined his practice to diseases of the eye, ear, nose, and throat, and was probably Lexington's first specialist. Dr. William L. Elmore, a native of Jessamine County whose medical career reached far into the twentieth century, became widely known in the city and nearby counties as a "baby doctor." He advised overburdened and overprotective young mothers to "put that baby on the ground" and also to "give that baby a drink of water. Don't you know babies get thirsty?" One patient believed Elmore to be a great physician because, though dispensing little medicine, he prescribed common sense in enormous doses.[27]

In welcoming physicians from across the Commonwealth to Lexington for the annual meeting of the Kentucky State Medical Association in May 1904, a prominent local attorney recalled the medical practitioner of his childhood. The old-time doctor, he said, gave ipecac and castor oil and, while awaiting results, took the knife he cut his plug tobacco with and measured out about 20 grains of calomel. No doubt the physicians laughed at his story which measured, at least in part, the distance traveled in medical practice during the nineteenth century.

4

MEDICAL PUBLICATIONS AND PROFESSIONAL SOCIETIES

Kentucky medical publications in the nineteenth century, excluding a large body of purely scientific and technical literature, played an important role in bringing some knowledge of medicine to the layman and in serving as media for professional communication. Certain books were well received by the reading public and brought their authors profitable returns. Medical journals were also commercial enterprises, being owned and operated by their editors who were usually members of medical school faculties. As such the journals tended to be personal vehicles and partisans of their editors' schools as well as forums for medical thought and debate.

The first Kentucky medical book, *American Medical Guide for the Use of Families*, by Dr. Thomas W. Ruble, was printed at Richmond in 1810. It is believed that proceeds from the book enabled Dr. Ruble to move to Louisville, where he announced the opening of a practice five years later. Shortly after settling near Versailles about 1815, Richard Carter, the noted "Indian doctor," published a book entitled *Valuable Vegetable*

Medical Prescriptions, for the Cure of All Nervous and Putrid Disorders. The second edition, printed in 1825, contains a mixture of herbal recipes, pious sayings, backwoods tall tales, and doggerel poems on subjects ranging from wedding night ecstasies to "the lamb of God." Claiming that "arbitrary custom and ignorant prejudice" were obstacles to a proper understanding of herbal medicine, Carter maintained that "the slightest reasoning drawn from real observation may be of more utility, and may give greater information to a judicious inquirer, than the most extensive theory produces, drawn from hypothesis alone."[1] This successful book helped its author to become well known as a botanic practitioner.

Unquestionably the most widely used home medical manual of the West and South was written by a Virginia-born regular physician, John C. Gunn, who moved from Tennessee to Louisville in 1838. *Gunn's Domestic Medicine or Poor Man's Friend*, first published in 1830, went through an untold number of editions for more than forty years and provided its author with a comfortable livelihood. He believed in treating illness with "good judgment and common sense," adding that "a long practice in my profession has fully convinced me that more favorable results take place from simple remedies, and good nursing, than from eminent physicians who quarrel with each other for pre-eminence in fame, instead of endeavoring to enlighten and advance the happiness of the human family."[2] Throughout the nineteenth century Dr. Gunn's book could be found in many Kentucky homes on a shelf next to the family Bible.

Two short-lived publications, which were not medical journals in the usual sense, may be mentioned briefly. In 1829 Anthony Hunn, the well-known Thomsonian practitioner who lived in Mercer County near Danville, began publishing *Medical Friend of the People* through which he attacked regular medicine, extolled Thomson's preparations, and advertised for students. In addition to botanic medicine Hunn offered to teach Romance languages, German, Greek, as well as piano, Spanish and Italian guitars, and, finally, "the art of fencing with the small sword, of which, by diploma, he is master."[3]

Two other Thomsonian physicians named Clapp and Lewis owned a botanical pharmacy, operated an infirmary, and published a similar journal, the *Western Botanic Recorder*, in Louisville in 1835.

The first Kentucky medical journal, the *Transylvania Journal of Medicine and the Associate Sciences*, edited by John Esten Cooke and Charles Wilkins Short, appeared in 1828. Lunsford P. Yandell became editor in 1832, and five years later he was succeeded by Robert Peter before suspension of publication in 1838. An attempt to revive the journal in 1849 under the name *Transylvania Medical Journal* lasted but two years. The *Kentucky Medical Recorder*, probably the successor to the *Transylvania Medical Journal*, appeared in Louisville from 1851 to 1854 in connection with the establishment of the Kentucky School of Medicine, but it ceased publication when the Transylvania faculty returned permanently to Lexington.

The most important journal of the period, the *Western Journal of Medicine and Surgery*, began in 1840 under the editorship of Daniel Drake and Lunsford P. Yandell. Over the years it compared favorably with the best medical publications in the United States. Another promising journal, the *Louisville Review: A Bi-Monthly Journal of Practical Medicine and Surgery*, was announced in 1856, but its editor and proprietor, Samuel D. Gross, took it to Philadelphia the next year. The *Louisville Medical Journal*, claiming to be affiliated with no group or school, made a short-lived appearance in 1860. After the Civil War, Edwin S. Gaillard edited the *Richmond and Louisville Medical Journal* for many years, and David W. Yandell (son of Lunsford P. Yandell) edited the *American Practitioner*, which had a long run and lasted into the twentieth century.

The journals commonly contained original articles, reports of unusual cases, and notices and reviews. They also tended to reflect the personality and outlook of their editors. Lunsford P. Yandell, for example, was a pious churchman who believed affinity for strong drink was the medical profession's besetting sin. As editor of the *Transylvania Journal of Medicine and the*

Associate Sciences in 1832 he published an article by his mentor, Charles Caldwell, condemning the traditional hospitality that induced doctors to take a drink for purposes of refreshment. With "the decanter, water-pitcher, and tumblers . . . as constant on the sideboard, as the sun is on his path" in many Lexington homes, physicians refreshed themselves to intoxication during a day's calls.[4] After moving to Louisville, Yandell bore most of the editorial duties of the *Western Journal of Medicine and Surgery*. A forceful writer himself, he dipped his pen in honey or gall according to the occasion.

Edwin S. Gaillard began publication of the *Richmond and Louisville Medical Journal* in 1868 with a review of a rival's work, an exercise he compared to stripping the "skin from an ass, and particularly from an old ass."[5] Yet however arrogant he may have been, Gaillard held strong journalistic principles. In 1871 he received a communication from Dr. Edward O. Guerrant of Mount Sterling describing the case of a young child who had swallowed a marble. Local physicians, including Guerrant's partner, ignored his belief that the marble had lodged in a bronchial passage and repeatedly dosed the child with calomel and castor oil. Postmortem examination brought tragic confirmation of Guerrant's diagnosis. He was at first reluctant to identify the other physicians, but Gaillard urged him to name them and let the chips fall where they might. That fall the *Richmond and Louisville Medical Journal* carried a full account of the case which strongly implied that Guerrant's associates were culpable of incompetence and malpractice.

Rivalry between medical schools was frequently accentuated by partisan warfare in the journals. When Gaillard became dean of both the Louisville Medical College and the Kentucky School of Medicine in 1875, he sought to advance their interests through a smaller publication, the *American Medical Weekly*. In January 1876, Richard O. Cowling and William H. Galt of the University of Louisville Medical Department launched the *Louisville Medical News* in a frontal attack on Gaillard and the LMC-KSM "phenomenon." At one point in the verbal slugfest Cowling and Galt called Gaillard to repentance and issued an ultimatum: (1) to choose between the Louisville Medical College and the Kentucky School of Medicine; (2) to discontinue the "beneficiary" fee scheme or make it honest; and (3) to stop graduating students with M.D. degrees after only nine months of study. Gaillard replied: "If a couple of boys armed with urethral syringes were to appear before the garrison of Gibraltar and send in their 'ultimatum,' the act could not be as ludicrous as the 'ultimatum,' of the [*Louisville Medical News*] . . . to the Louisville Medical College." Feigning shock at such a coarse rejoinder, Cowling and Galt "respectfully suggested that, in view of the nature of the Gibraltar we are besieging, *rectal* syringes would be 'conspicuously' more 'appropriate.' "[6] This was one of the rare occasions on which Gaillard's adversaries bested him in an encounter.

Prior to the 1870s efforts to achieve professional objectives in Kentucky through the formation of medical societies invariably resulted in failure. At the time of the Revolution basic professional objectives of newly formed medical societies included promotion of harmony among qualified practitioners through association and through adherence to uniform fee schedules. More important, the societies sought to distinguish between qualified and unqualified practitioners through educational requirements and to license the former by examination. In most states by 1800 there was evidence of progress toward these goals, but between 1820 and 1850 the situation changed dramatically. During these years most older states repealed their licensing statutes and newer states failed to adopt any at all. Two developments were most important in bringing about this change: the rapid growth of proprietary medical schools, which graduated an ever-increasing number of young men with M.D. degrees, and the appearance of bitterly competitive groups of sectarian practitioners. Even in old, established Philadelphia, doctors "lived in an almost constant state of warfare,—quarreling, and even worse, was not uncommon among them, and now and then street fights occurred." Another observer of the times noted, "If we look for the effect of a restless, ambitious spirit, we shall nowhere see it more manifest than in a densely populated place, where a number of physicians are brought into the same neighborhood."[7] Under these conditions the older state medical societies collapsed and attempts by regular physicians to form local societies were usually abortive.

The first Kentucky medical organization, the Lexington Medical Society, was formed in the winter of 1799/1800 by apprentices of the town's half dozen regular physicians, who were made honorary members. Strengthened by the beginning of full medical instruction at Transylvania in 1817, this first society later became closely related to the Kentucky Medical Society of Transylvania University, an alumni group. About 1820 Dr. Samuel Brown, then professor of the theory and practice of medicine, organized the Kappa Lambda Society of Hippocrates among Transylvania medical students. A secret fraternity, its purpose was to promote unity and harmony in the profession, and initiates pledged themselves to a strict code of ethics.

Writing in 1819 Dr. Henry McMurtrie, Louisville's first historian, stated that twenty-two physicians were engaged in practice there. In February of that year fifteen of them, including William C. Galt, Thomas Booth, and Richard Ferguson, publicly announced the formation of a medical society for purposes of scientific advancement and establishment of a fee schedule. Unfortunately, neither the name they adopted nor the fee schedule has survived. Almost twenty years later, in 1838, the General Assembly chartered two medical societies: the Louisville Medical Society and the College of Physicians and Surgeons of the City of Louisville. The histories of these early societies are relatively obscure, but the former was sponsored by the faculty of the newly established Louisville Medical Institute while the latter may have been composed chiefly of physicians who opposed the medical school. In any case both societies eventually suffered the fate of two other short-lived groups, the Louisville District Medical Society, formed in 1841, and the Louisville Academy of Medicine, established the following year. By the Civil War period all had fallen

44

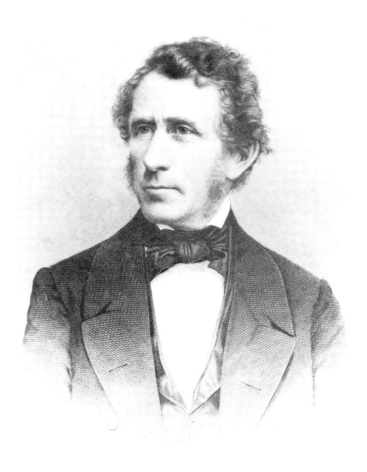

Daniel Drake, M.D. (1785–1852)

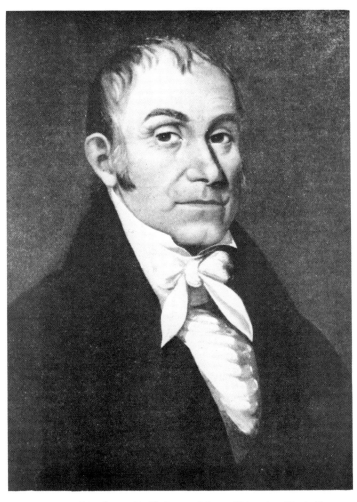

Courtesy of Kornhauser Health Sciences Library, University of Louisville

Ephraim McDowell, M.D. (1771–1830)

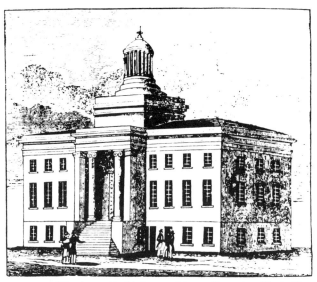

Louisville Medical Institute, 1838

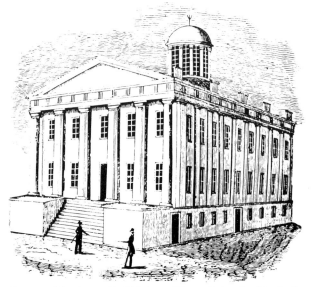

Transylvania Medical Hall, 1840

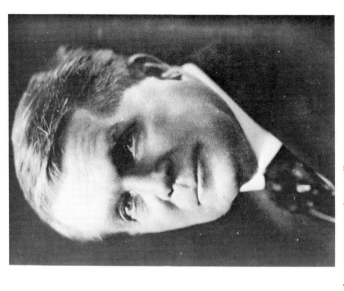

Joseph N. McCormack, M.D. (1847–1922)

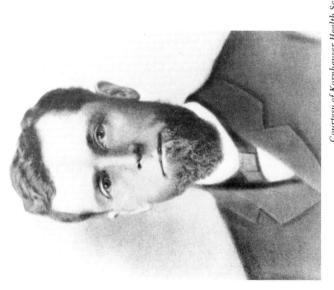

Robert B. Pusey, M.D. (1836–1889)

Courtesy of Kornhauser Health Sciences Library, University of Louisville

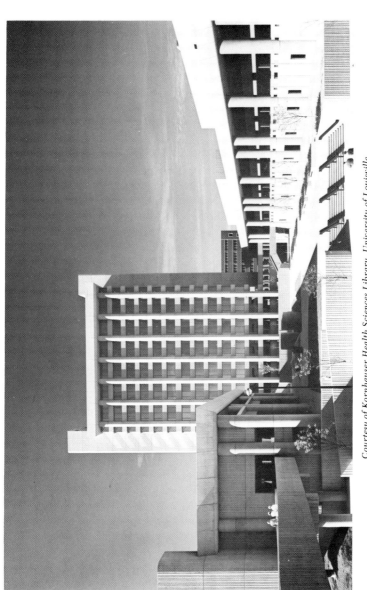

Courtesy of Kornhauser Health Sciences Library, University of Louisville

Health Sciences Center, University of Louisville, 1975

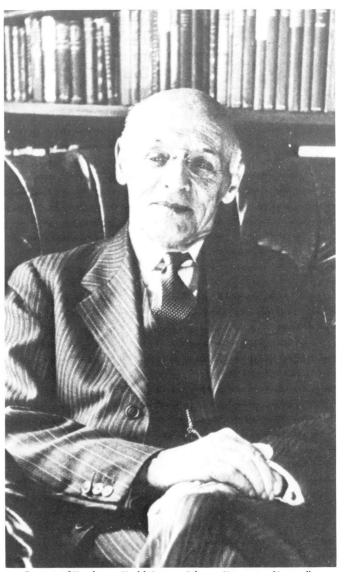

Abraham Flexner (1866–1959)

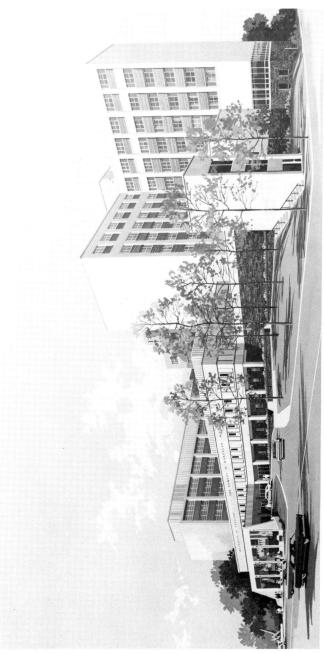

Albert B. Chandler Medical Center, University of Kentucky

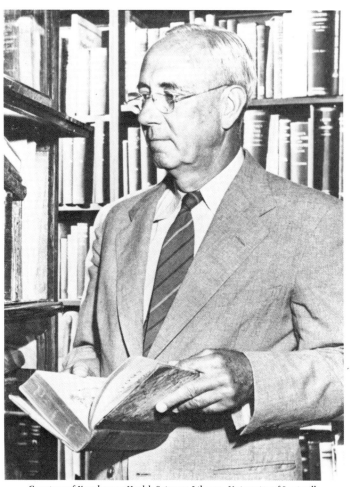

Emmet Field Horine, M.D. (1885–1964)

apart, mainly because of factional controversies and strife. The earliest local society still in existence, the Medico-Chirurgical Society of Louisville, was organized by Dr. Edwin S. Gaillard and thirteen other physicians on November 21, 1868.

Relations between physicians in Lexington were very likely at low ebb in March 1831, when Charles Caldwell, professor of the institutes of medicine and physiology at Transylvania, gave a lecture to the Lexington Medical Society on professional behavior. In his view the physician should strive to cultivate the manners of a gentleman without affectation and avoid the company of "bacchanalian revellers." He should seek a full knowledge of medicine, be busy in his work, and also avoid the entanglements of politics and religion. Exhibition of a modest civic spirit in behalf of public improvements, particularly education, brought good to the community and enhanced the doctor's reputation. But of all things most injurious, said Caldwell, "is the want of harmony and concert" within the profession. "*E pluribus unum*, is a motto as essential in defence of professional truth and character, as in defence of confederated states. But it is a motto to which, as a body, physicians are strangers." Remedy for the evil, he believed, might be had through "union, gentlemanly harmony, and concert in action among the members of the profession. Thus will the strength of all become, in some degree, the strength of each one . . . , a solid fabric, which nothing can shake." Anticipating the formation of the American Medical Association by sixteen years, Caldwell advocated the organization of state medical societies to gather vital statistics, acquaint physicians with one another, and regulate practice by a standard code of ethics. A national "Diet, or Amphyctyonic Council," might then be set up to "superintend the interests of the whole."[8]

A representative picture of early Kentucky medical societies emerges from the pages of a surviving minute book. On December 9, 1835, sixteen physicians met at the Phoenix Hotel to organize the College of Physicians and Surgeons of Lexington. Dr. Robert C. Holland addressed the gathering as did Professors Caldwell and William H. Richardson from the medical college. Then, on motion of Dr. Caleb W. Cloud, the group appointed a committee on organization. During three subsequent meetings, including one on February 1, 1836, when the first president, Dr. Caldwell, gave an inaugural address in Transylvania's Medical Hall, the founders adopted both a constitution and regulatory by-laws. Twenty-three physicians signed the charter granted February 25; five new members were elected in 1837; and, among this membership, the majority were either Transylvania medical faculty or alumni.

The College of Physicians and Surgeons sought "to advance the Science of medicine" by observation and study, to share these researches with each other during regular meetings the first Tuesday of every month, thereby "cultivating and cherishing order and uniformity in the performance of the practical duties of the profession." Candidates for membership must be "practitioners of medicine and Surgery of acknowledged attainment and good moral standing" residing in Lexington or Fayette County, although the residence restriction was soon lifted to include the entire state of Kentucky. The society's by-laws required prior announcement of papers or subjects of discussion to be presented at each meeting, and it was the specified duty of members "to encourage Post Mortem examinations." One standing committee was appointed to keep a meteorological register, and another was obliged to record prevailing diseases and report at meetings. Finally, the by-laws provided that "Percival's System of Medical Ethics shall be the guide of each member of the College in his professional intercourse and moral deportment."[9] There was no mention whatever of a standard fee schedule.

By limiting membership to physicians "of acknowledged attainment," the Lexington adherents of regular or orthodox medicine attempted to distinguish themselves from other sectarian practitioners, whom they regarded as both enemies and quacks. Within two years of its founding, however, the society was practically defunct. No doubt the blowup at Transylvania in 1837, when half the medical faculty moved to Louisville, aroused partisan antagonisms. At the meeting of November 7 that year one member proposed to amend the by-laws so that "any member failing to comply with the requisitions of the constitution, or who shall be guilty of any immorality whatsoever unbecoming a gentleman shall be subject to expulsion from the College." In 1838 and again in 1839, on request of the mayor and city council, members were assigned to attend inmates of the City Hospital and Work House. But during these years a quorum of five was rarely present at monthly meetings. On December 3, 1839, the college adjourned, having scheduled a meeting for the first Tuesday in January, 1840; yet it did not convene again until July 16, 1846. No quorum was present at the next meeting, April 2, 1850. On April 5 three members holding proxies from three others gathered to elect new members and then adjourned to meet April 16 for the purpose of nominating delegates to the American Medical Association convention in Cincinnati. But apparently the local meeting never took place.

Amid competition, conflict, and declining economic status, leaders of the nation's medical profession had met in Philadelphia in 1847 to organize the American Medical Association. The delegates believed professional problems could be resolved by bringing doctors together, interesting them in scientific pursuits such as the recording of vital statistics, promoting harmony and unity through a code of ethics, and by effecting certain reforms in medical education. Four years later, in 1851, the General Assembly enacted laws incorporating the Kentucky State Medical Society and requiring that county records of births and deaths be kept. The thirty-five incorporators and subsequently elected members formally endorsed the AMA code of ethics and called for the formation of county medical societies. They also began annual publication of the society's *Transactions*, one of the more significant nineteenth-century Kentucky medical imprints.

At its inception, however, and for many years afterward, the state medical society was sharply divided on the issue of educational reform, a question that touched the economic interests both of medical school professors and of community practitioners. In 1850 Kentucky had 1,470 doctors in a population of 982,405, a ratio of 1:688. Dr. William L. Sutton of

Georgetown in Scott County, a founder of the society and "the father of vital statistics" in Kentucky, believed that professional decline had come about through an excess production of medical school graduates "armed with diplomas." Many of them were so ignorant, said Sutton, that they could not "tell whether or not a woman has a prostate gland." The resulting competition for practice produced an effect comparable to Gresham's law. "It is said that competition is the life of trade. It is all very well within certain limits. But," Sutton added, "when more goods are manufactured than can be consumed, the value of each parcel is lessened, and some must remain unsold. The best samples, being higher priced, must first be driven from the market."[10]

Medical school professors took a different view of the AMA's proposals for reform, which included extending the course of study and requiring schools to provide clinical instruction. With its enrollments already declining, such measures would have driven Transylvania to the wall. Referring to AMA conventions as "the annual [S]anhedrin," Dr. Robert Peter, a member of both the Transylvania faculty and the state medical society, argued that the principles of medicine and clinical teaching were distinct and separate spheres, the one preparatory to the other. Clinical instruction at the expense of basic knowledge, he said, "can only result in the production of routine quack-salvers."[11] Peter believed that the Kentucky profession's fundamental problem was lack of a state law regulating medical practice by providing for licensure.

By the 1870s, as the state medical society recovered from the dislocations of the Civil War, there were an estimated 5,000 practitioners in the Commonwealth, of whom about 1,000 had either never attended medical school or had not graduated. Also at this time, according to a later president of the society, Dr. Lewis S. McMurtry of Louisville, "The cities were infested with advertising charlatans and the traveling nostrum vendors traversed the country, imposing upon the credulity of the people and filching their money."[12] These conditions, combined with a growing professional sentiment favoring reform in medical education, resulted in state medical society sponsorship of legislation passed by the General Assembly in 1874 under the title "AN ACT to protect citizens of this Commonwealth from Empiricism."

By the provisions of Kentucky's first licensing law a board of medical examiners in each judicial district was to determine the fitness of every practitioner by examination in chemistry, anatomy, physiology, obstetrics, surgery, and practical medicine. Doctors holding diplomas from chartered medical colleges and those "regularly and honorably engaged in practice for ten years" were exempt. Applicants for examination had to present evidence of good moral character and pay a fee of twenty dollars in order to obtain a license valid for not less than one year nor more than five. Practitioners violating the law were subject to a fine of fifty dollars on first conviction and one hundred dollars and thirty days, either or both, on subsequent convictions. Since the examining boards consisted of five "regular graduates," and those "regularly" engaged in practice for ten years were exempted, it appears that the state medical society intended to use strong medicine on sectarian competitors who were not medical school graduates.

During the following decade a few permanent county medical societies were established with Boyle, Hardin, and Fayette being among the first. At the same time Dr. Joseph N. McCormack, secretary of the Kentucky State Board of Health (established in 1878) and also a leader of the state medical society, sought to bring the society into close relation with the state government, as Dr. Jerome Cochran had done in Alabama. Under McCormack's leadership the medical practice act was amended in 1887 by requiring physicians to register their diplomas from state or other "reputable" medical colleges with county clerks. A further amendment in 1893 vested the State Board of Health with both licensing power and authority to control professional behavior. The new law provided for licensing of any physician with an acceptable diploma, or of the regular practitioner lacking a degree who could show satisfactory evidence of reputable practice prior to February 23, 1864. It prohibited the "itinerant doctor" from either registering or practicing. Section 5 stated: "The State Board of Health may refuse to issue the certificate provided for in section three of this article to any individual guilty of grossly unprofessional conduct . . . and it may, after due notice and hearing, revoke such certificates for like cause." During the period 1888–1893 approximately 1,200 physicians either quit practice or left the state.

At the turn of the century, however, the majority of Kentucky physicians still belonged to no medical society, and professional relations were characterized by bitter competition and conflict among and between regulars and other sectarian practitioners, notably homeopaths and the newly emerging sect of osteopathy. In the years to come Dr. McCormack would provide further leadership in a search for solutions to professional problems.

5

REFORM AND RECONSTRUCTION

No TWO MEN have had an impact on the American medical profession and its institutions comparable to that of two Kentuckians, one a physician and the other a schoolteacher. Born on a Nelson County farm November 9, 1847, Joseph Nathaniel McCormack was mostly self-taught as a boy, learning while working with his brothers and their farmer-storekeeper father. After graduating from the Miami Medical College of Ohio in 1870, he returned to Nelson County, married, and began the practice of medicine. McCormack encountered difficulties, however, including a severe illness with typhoid fever, and in 1876 he moved to Bowling Green in Warren County to join the practice of an elderly physician, Dr. Lemuel C. Porter. Outstanding service during the Bowling Green yellow fever epidemic in 1878 brought him an appointment to the State Board of Health the following year. As its secretary and executive officer after 1883, McCormack designed Kentucky's increasingly restrictive medical practice laws and sought legislation to advance the cause of public health.

McCormack's success in mixing politics and medicine, his reorganizational work in the Kentucky State Medical Society, and his magnetic personality brought him to the attention of high officials in the American Medical Association who sought to make that organization an effective force in national politics.

At the turn of the century fewer than 9,000 of the country's approximately 100,000 regular physicians held membership in the AMA, and no more than 25 percent belonged to affiliated state and local societies. Moreover, since 40 percent of doctors who had a direct or indirect relationship to the AMA lived in a cluster of states contiguous to its Chicago headquarters, the organization was really a northcentral and eastern regional medical society with little or no influence in the South and West. R. L. Polk's *Medical and Surgical Register of the United States* for 1890 lists twenty-three state, sectarian, specialty, and local medical societies in Kentucky. At that time the state medical society scarcely enrolled 10 percent of the Commonwealth's approximately 3,000 regular physicians. By 1903, with its name changed that year, the Kentucky State Medical Association had enrolled nearly 1,400 regular doctors, thanks to Dr. McCormack's decade of organizational work.

Appointed chairman of the AMA's Committee on Organization in 1900, McCormack's design for reform was adopted the following year. One object of the plan was to bring doctors who had strayed into specialty organizations back into the general fold. A second closely related object was to make the county medical society the profession's basic organizational unit. Local membership automatically conferred membership in the state medical society, and state societies were constituent members of the AMA. Where Dr. Charles Caldwell had envisioned a "Diet" or "Amphyctyonic Council" to rule the whole in 1831, McCormack's committee placed legislative power in the hands of representatives from state societies to be known as the AMA's House of Delegates. In 1903, as a further effort to swell the ranks of organized medicine, the AMA abandoned the old ethical code's sanctions against professional relations with other sectarian practitioners. By the terms of a new statement of principles any licensed physician, whatever his educational background, who would not "designate" or label his method of practice would be received into full fellowship, including medical society membership, by his regular brethren.

In Kentucky, the annual meeting of the KSMA got under way

in Louisville on April 22, 1903, with announcements by the local arrangements chairman of a smoker, compliments of the Jefferson County Medical Society, and a hospitality visit to the Fehr Brewing Company. Doctors could take streetcars to the brewery, said the chairman, "and we will arrange to have patrol wagons and ambulances to bring you back."[1] But the association, dominated as was the State Board of Health by McCormack's forceful leadership, had more serious business also. After McCormack called on the membership to pledge support to incoming officers and to association councillors, who would visit counties either to establish or to invigorate local medical societies, the president, Dr. W. W. Richmond, of Clinton, elaborated the goals of organization in his address. With seventy county societies represented in the House of Delegates, Dr. F. H. Gaines of Carroll County offered a resolution urging KSMA support for revision of Kentucky's medical practice law by acting "at once, and as one man, for the accomplishment of the end desired."[2] McCormack drafted the new law, approved by the legislature March 18, 1904, to conform to the AMA's 1903 statement of principles. By its provisions the State Board of Health was reorganized to consist of eight physicians: five regulars, one homeopath, one eclectic, and one osteopath. Five of these, two regulars and the other sectarians, constituted an examining committee. The board itself had authority to grant medical licenses, or it could refuse and revoke them for cause including "chronic or persistent inebriety . . . or other grossly unprofessional or dishonorable conduct."[3]

As the AMA's chief of organization, McCormack traveled the length and breadth of the land between 1902 and 1912, speaking to audiences of physicians and laymen in virtually every county in the nation. His main objective was to raise medicine's economic, social, and political status through a grassroots organizational movement. At the same time he appealed for a reform coalition of laymen and doctors who, by working together, could best serve the interests of society by first serving those of the profession. During his campaign McCormack served as an advance agent for solicitors from the AMA's

Chicago headquarters who then worked with state medical society district councillors to enlist licensed physicians into
county medical societies. Once organized, the local societies
were to be supervised by councillors who had responsibility
for professional discipline.

A strikingly handsome man and a gifted orator, McCormack
combined down-home phrases and biblical metaphor to de-
liver a shrewd message in evangelical style on the business of
medicine that was all the more disarming for its recital of professional sins. In two speeches he gave hundreds of times,
"Organization and Its Advantages to the Individual Doctor,"
and "What the People Should Know about the Doctors and
What the Doctors Should Know about Themselves," McCormack berated physicians for running their affairs "like a widow
woman runs a farm."[4] Eroded by inflation, the average physician's income had declined since the 1890s, and many were
barely able to support their families, much less keep abreast of
developments in medicine. Moreover, isolation and segrega-
tion relegated many doctors to the periphery of the profession.
Since modern, responsible communities owed their citizens
first-class medical care, laymen should see that physicians received adequate compensation, and they should also support
active county medical societies. Through the latter, doctors
could obtain continuing education by harmonious sharing of
scientific knowledge.

Fundamentally, however, McCormack believed medicine's
degraded economic and social status and almost utter lack of
political influence was an internal professional problem.
Long-standing envies, jealousies, backbitings, and an almost
constitutional inability to agree with another doctor had
sapped public confidence and esteem that must be regained.
In his speeches he repeatedly cited the conflicts among the
Louisville medical schools. Earlier, he said, he had thought
the spirit of medical strife and enmity was confined to Kentucky. But he found it everywhere, a sore on the body of
medicine as preventable as typhoid fever. It could and must
be stopped by bringing doctors together in a fraternal spirit of

professional accord. To McCormack and other AMA leaders, this was what medical organization was all about.

In later years McCormack remembered that "probably never before did a reform so sweep a profession, and now, regardless of schools or pathies, ours is rapidly becoming one of the most harmonious of callings."[5] But the reform movement did not proceed unchallenged or unopposed. After enactment of the Kentucky medical practice law in 1904, which admitted other sectarian practitioners to equal standing with regular physicians, some doctors in Covington raised the standard of revolt, declaring their independence of the Campbell-Kenton County Medical Society, the third largest in the state. Calling for organization of medical societies that would return to the old code of ethics, they charged the AMA with sacrificing ethics to greed. Dominated by specialists "blinded by the almighty dollar," the national organization had abandoned traditional ethical precepts to enlarge the field of consultation. The Covington doctors proposed to uphold the honor of traditional medicine and to resist efforts to lower the profession to the level of a trade.[6] But they were no match for the force of reform.

A man with less missionary zeal or physical stamina than McCormack could hardly have endured the schedule he kept up for ten years. Usually state medical society journals prepared the way for his visits, as did the *Kentucky Medical Journal* beginning in January 1906. Its editor (McCormack's son, Dr. Arthur T. McCormack) urged Kentucky doctors "to search our hearts and purge them of any envious and censorious monsters which may have found lodgment there." The April issue carried McCormack's itinerary from April 30 to May 26, 1906, during which he made thirty-eight speeches, on fourteen occasions speaking in two different towns the same day. Local medical society members were urged to support the events by inviting farmers, businessmen, lawyers, teachers, "the ladies," and particularly those doctors who had not yet been "called." By plain talk McCormack would provide "insight into the very heart of things," wielding a verbal "shillalah" with the same grace he used in applying unguental balm. Some listeners might "go out with heads a little sore," but all would be "better in heart for having heard."[7]

Where possible, state medical society officers participated in the meetings, especially the district councillors who were responsible for organizing doctors at the county level. One Kentucky councillor, Dr. James G. Carpenter of Stanford in Lincoln County, believed his work required obedience to Jesus' command to "go to the uttermost parts of the earth." Advertising his coming by newspaper, Carpenter would then write the doctors personal letters: "I am going to organize a society, and I am going to get you in good standing, in the bond of fellowship and love. I will stay until my money gives out, and I will stay among the brethren free of charge. I have come to settle the troubles, and by the grace of God they are going to be settled, and I will bring the doctors into the fold."[8] McCormack himself likened the councillor's role to that of a bishop; both functions were essentially pastoral. For example, he told a meeting in 1911, if the physicians in Bullitt County failed to meet regularly and on time, the councillor should write each one announcing his coming at a time and place and then telephone one doctor to have dinner ready. But, Dr. Charles Z. Aud of Cecilian in Hardin County asked, what if the county medical society's secretary stated that local doctors were tending to their business and suggested that the councillor do the same? "I would not pay any attention to that," McCormack replied. "That secretary needs a bishop."[9]

By 1909, according to the *American Medical Directory*, or about two years before McCormack's retirement from active organizational work, 2,149 of the Commonwealth's 3,708 licensed physicians were subject to professional discipline by state and local organizations. Yet there were few constraints on the portals to the profession—the medical schools, which in the United States and Canada numbered 155 at that time. From the beginning McCormack's speeches alluded to a need for reconstruction in medical education, and in 1907 the AMA's Council on Medical Education named Louisville as one of "five especially rotten spots" in the nation. No doubt such adverse publicity, combined with hard times, was a factor in the merger of Louisville Medical College with the Hospital College of Medicine and the consolidation of Kentucky University Medical Department with the University of Louisville Medical Department that year. In 1908 all the old regular schools, except the Louisville National Medical College for blacks, merged with the University of Louisville. But the process of educational reform was not yet complete.

Born in Louisville in 1866, the sixth child of German immigrant parents, Abraham Flexner spent his early childhood in the period known as Reconstruction. His father, a small merchant who was wiped out by the Panic of 1873, died in 1882, leaving the family to struggle under the double burdens of poverty and anti-Semitism. Flexner recalled that "his ideals were his legacy—his only legacy—to his family." The Louisville of Abraham's childhood days was a bustling river city of 150,000, with a "quite distinctly stratified" society ruled by a proud upper crust who "lived beyond their means, smoked, drank, gambled, used a revolver frequently on slight provocation, and made Louisville what it still is, the racing center of the western hemisphere." Young Flexner also despised the aristocratic pretensions of Lexington and the Bluegrass where inhabitants "cultivated courtly manners, and in a vague way felt themselves lords of creation." Moritz and Esther Flexner were pious Jews, attending synagogue and observing feasts all their lives, but their children rejected this heritage. "For us," wrote Flexner, "Herbert Spencer and Huxley, then at the height of their fame and influence, replaced the Bible and the prayer book."[10]

With the help of his older brother Jacob, a pharmacist, Abraham attended Johns Hopkins University in 1884, graduating two years later with an A.B. degree at the age of nineteen. A poor boy, poorly prepared, his preliminary examinations in classics were unsatisfactory, but kindly professors gave him extra help to overcome deficiencies. This experience led him to believe that "a half-taught boy, bitterly aware of the fact," who could keep quiet, learn, and constantly strive to join the company of his superiors, had a brighter future than more fortunate lads. "Such, at any rate," he wrote in 1940, "was the conviction I soon reached at Baltimore and still maintain."[11]

After graduation, Flexner returned home in 1886 to teach at Louisville High School for four years while supporting his mother. In 1889 his brother Simon received an M.D. degree from "one of the wretched schools that then flourished," the Medical Department of the University of Louisville, which also granted their brother Jacob an honorary M.D. on May 15, 1894. Feeling a need for more income, Abraham opened a private school for boys in 1890, "Mr. Flexner's School," whose patrons were Louisville's upper crust. In teaching their sons, he wrote, "I pushed those who showed aptitude for a given subject and was patient where no aptitude existed." Perhaps like professors in proprietary medical colleges his "bread and butter depended on succeeding with stupid or indifferent pupils," but "then as now at heart I really cared about excellence."[12]

The schoolmaster's reputation brought a request from John M. Atherton, a distiller and one of Louisville's richest men, to tutor his niece, Anne Laziere Crawford, the great-granddaughter of an 1824 presidential candidate, for entrance to Vassar. Romance bloomed in this student-teacher relationship, and after Anne graduated from college the couple married in June 1898. Seven years later Flexner closed his school and, with his wife and six-year-old daughter, went to Cambridge to begin graduate studies in psychology at Harvard. Soon, however, like many Americans of that day, he was drawn to the German universities in a quest for scientific learning and, perhaps, in search of his own cultural roots. The Flexners arrived in Berlin during the fall of 1906, and during the next two years he attended lectures and wrote a book, *The American College: A Criticism*, which unfavorably compared American universities with those of Germany. Following the book's publication in 1908, with financial resources depleted, the family returned to New York where Flexner applied for a job to Dr. Henry S. Pritchett, an astronomer and former president of the Massachusetts Institute of Technology, at that time president of the newly established Carnegie Foundation for the Advancement of Teaching. Pritchett asked if he would do a study of medical schools along the lines of his book on American colleges. "About December 1, 1908," Flexner remembered later, "I set to work on my survey of medical education in the United States and Canada."[13]

At first Flexner had doubts about his qualifications to undertake such a study. Not only did he lack training in medicine but, he told Pritchett, he had never even so much as "set my foot inside a medical school." Pritchett assuaged his doubts, assuring him this was all to the good since the task required a mind free from the prejudice of medical knowledge. With guidance from his brother Simon, then director of the Rockefeller Medical Institute, and from Dr. William H. Welch and other members of the Johns Hopkins medical faculty, Flexner's qualms were laid to rest. Throughout the study he worked closely with AMA secretary Dr. George H. Simmons, and Dr. N. P. Colwell of the AMA's Council on Medical Education traveled with him on visits to schools. Having such assistance Flexner could make "a reliable estimate" of any medical school in just "a few hours."[14] Completed in little more than a year, the study was published in 1910 as Bulletin Number 4 of the prestigious Carnegie Foundation for the Advancement of Teaching under the title *Medical Education in the United States and Canada.*

In an introductory summary Dr. Pritchett stated Flexner's salient findings. Since the 1880s medical schools had produced an overwhelming number of poorly trained doctors, in utter disregard of public welfare, to the point that the United States had four to five times more physicians in proportion to population than Germany. This overproduction was perpetrated primarily by commercial schools that used advertising methods to divert "a mass of unprepared youth" from industrial occupations into medicine. Most of these schools had failed to keep pace with the movement of medical instruction from the lecture room to the laboratory because of the increased costs of the new facilities and declining school incomes. The schools' defense that they offered opportunity to "the poor boy" was unacceptable; a reputable medical school must have the highest curriculum standards, professors dedicated to clinical science, and a teaching hospital under full educational control. The adduced facts of the report made it clear, wrote Pritchett, that the interests of American society would be best served by limiting the supply of doctors.

Flexner acknowledged the trend since 1904 toward a decline in numbers of schools and graduates; the problem at hand was "to calculate how far tendencies already observable may be carried without harm." In 1910 Kentucky had 3,708 physicians in a population estimated at 2,406,859, for a ratio of 1:649. This overcrowding of the profession, Flexner wrote, was exemplified by Henderson County (1:624) where a practitioner could be found within five miles of any point. Since most of these were graduates of Louisville schools, there could be no doubt that "Kentucky is one of the largest producers of low-grade doctors in the entire Union."[15]

The culprits in this disservice to the Commonwealth and nation were, or at least had been, Louisville's regular schools "to which crude boys thronged from the plantations." Apparently forgetting his own background, Flexner believed the argument in behalf of schools that offered opportunity to poor boys, poorly prepared, to be a specious one. Repeatedly using the word "reconstruction" throughout the report, he defined the purpose of medicine in an industrial social order: "The medical profession is a social organ, created not for the purpose of gratifying the inclinations or preferences of certain individuals, but as a means of promoting health, physical vigor, happiness—and the economic independence and efficiency immediately connected with these factors. Whether most men support themselves or become charges on the community depends on their keeping well, or if ill, promptly getting well. Now, can anyone seriously contend that in the midst of abundant educational resources, a congenial or profitable career in medicine is to be made for an individual regardless of his capacity to satisfy the purpose for which the profession exists? . . . Your 'poor boy' has no right, natural, indefeasible, or acquired, to enter upon the practice of medicine unless it is best for society that he should."[16]

Flexner believed that the number of medical schools could be reduced from 155 to 31 without depriving sections of the country capable of properly supporting them. Inadequate support meant low admission standards and unacceptably inferior education. The Southwestern Homeopathic Medical College and the Louisville National Medical College for blacks were among 56 schools having resources of less than $10,000 per year. With a staff of twenty-seven and a class of thirteen, the Louisville homeopathic school had an income of $1,100, and was, in Flexner's view, "utterly hopeless." In one room of its "filthy and neglected" building he found a bedraggled mannikin to be the sole means of instruction; "in another, a single guinea pig awaits his fate in a cage." The school's entrance requirements were reported to be the same as those of the University of Louisville Medical Department, but in another place Flexner stated that the homeopathic institution "cannot be said to have admission standards in any strict sense at all." Brief note of his visit to the Louisville National Medical College in January 1909 mentions less than high school requirement, faculty of twenty-three, class of forty, income of $2,560, and nominal laboratory facilities. However, he did observe that "a small and scrupulously clean hospital of 8 beds is connected with the school."[17]

At the time of Flexner's visit to the University of Louisville, a recent graduate of the old Kentucky School of Medicine, Emmet F. Horine, M.D., destined to become an eminent cardiologist and Kentucky's leading medical historian, had just been appointed assistant to the chairs of surgery, abdominal surgery, and gynecology. Flexner found admission standards low and poorly enforced, a class of 600, and a teaching staff of 90 in which professorships were heavily weighted toward surgery. He also reported that staff and teaching facilities for chemistry, pathology, bacteriology, physiology, and pharmacy, were desperately inadequate. Clinical teaching in the school's small hospital was all but impossible; the out-patient dispensary offered little more; and opportunities at City Hospital were limited to weekly amphitheater clinics for 100 to 300 students. The medical department's dependence on tuition fees for annual income of $75,125 kept admission requirements and educational standards low. UL students spent 220 of 450 instructional hours in didactic lectures, and Flexner believed the time devoted to quiz-drill memorization was completely wasted.

Summing up the Kentucky situation, and elaborating his social theory of medical education, Flexner condemned the Southwestern Homeopathic Medical College as a school "without merit" whose graduates deserved "no recognition whatsoever." Among seven medical schools for blacks in the country, the Louisville National Medical College was one of five that sent out "undisciplined men, whose lack of real training is covered up by the imposing M.D. degree." Flexner thought Meharry and Howard should be developed so "the more promising" blacks could "receive a substantial education in which hygiene rather than surgery, for example, is strongly accentuated." Such men would perceive that "duty calls them away from large cities to the village and the plantation, upon which light has hardly as yet begun to break." As with poor boys and blacks, Flexner also had a place for women. Earlier barriers in medical education had fallen before the Progressive Era's aggressive "New Woman." In view of this development, he believed the woman physician had an apparent function "in certain medical specialties" and that her "place in general medicine under some obvious limitations" was assured.[18]

Flexner considered the University of Louisville's prospects unpromising. Sources of support for the high standard in medical education set by Johns Hopkins were nowhere evident. The medical department was merely an amalgam of five old schools, and the university's newly established academic department was said to be unworthy of the name. Flexner claimed the state university in Lexington could not help since it had "never been an active educational factor" and now, with a politician as president, it floundered in "educational ineptitude."[19] In 1910 the *Journal of the American Medical As-*

sociation hailed the Carnegie report as a careful, objective study and, coming as it did from an independent agency, "it is sure to have a most profound influence on medical education in general, and claims of partiality or prejudice cannot be made against it."[20]

In the years immediately following the report's publication the once poor Jewish boy from Louisville (who eventually founded Princeton's Institute for Advanced Studies) was employed by the Rockefeller philanthropies, notably the General Education Board, which led the way in private foundation support for deserving medical schools. In order to obtain this support, an A rating from the AMA's Council on Medical Education was almost essential. Such a rating required strict adherence to educational standards, provision and maintenance of required instructional facilities, and small classes of medical students. In 1920 the University of Louisville admitted 44 freshmen into a total enrollment of 138 and conferred the M.D. degree on 25 graduates.

Such were the dimensions of reform and reconstruction in Kentucky medicine between 1900 and 1920. Taken together, the developments of this period constitute the most important episode in the social history of American medicine. By the time of President Warren G. Harding's inauguration, some of its implications for the Bluegrass state were already apparent.

6

PREVENTIVE MEDICINE AND PUBLIC HEALTH

Back in 1881, in his presidential address before the Kentucky State Medical Society in Covington, Dr. Lyman B. Todd of Lexington urged doctors to provide "that security which humanity demands" from preventable disease. The scene he envisioned in every community was one in which physicians, as friends and teachers, gathered families around each hearthstone to explain the principles of hygiene. As a result, "thousands of lives, now annually doomed to destruction, would be saved, and the health and comfort of the people greatly increased and secured."[1]

Forty years later, despite some evidence of progress, the need for private practice of preventive medicine was believed to be greater than ever. In 1900, for example, Kentucky had 3,538 deaths from tuberculosis, or 148.18 per 1,000 of total mortalities. That situation improved somewhat by 1920, but according to Dr. Will J. Shelton of Mayfield, in a paper presented before the state medical association meeting at Louisville in 1921, about 4,000 children were stricken with diphtheria each year of whom nearly 300 died. In rural areas, especially, typhoid fever remained a major disease problem, and Dr. Shelton urged physicians to concentrate on protective immunization for both diseases. It was a matter of professional interest to the general practitioner and to specialists that this course be pursued in a cooperative manner. Otherwise, he said, "there is a possibility of political control, or state medicine."[2]

Earlier, Dr. Todd had used the phrase "state medicine" interchangeably with preventive medicine as part of an argument for reducing traffic on the profession's highway by raising educational standards and, at the same time, acquiring power to selectively choose those fellow travelers best qualified to serve professional and public interests through medical licensure laws. These privileges and powers were obtained through the state, and by 1920 the profession had come to regard them as rights, although, as Dr. Shelton indicated, not without apprehensions about their source. The internal logic of Todd's concept of preventive medicine—a doctor at every fireside engaged in spreading the gospel of community hygiene—clearly called for expansion rather than restriction of the profession's numbers. However, the declining trend of the 1880s and 1890s continued as a result of professional reform and reconstruction. In 1909 Abraham Flexner found 3,708 licensed physicians in the Commonwealth and described Kentucky as medically overcrowded. By 1940 the number of doctors fell to 2,761; yet, in the interval, the state's population increased by almost 700,000.

The ideal of preventive medicine corresponded to no reality of private medical practice. And, since their livelihood seemed to depend on acute and chronic illnesses, most doctors feared preventive medicine was a path to the poorhouse. Speaking as a health officer and as a leader of organized medicine, Dr. Joseph N. McCormack sought to persuade physicians that their fears were unfounded. He repeatedly emphasized the relationship between preventive medicine, health education, and professional organization in a famous speech, "The New Gospel of Health and Long Life," given many times toward the end of his career. Dr. Shelton restated this theme in 1921 when he said: "Instead of lessening the work of physicians by preventing sickness you will increase the interest in the community and the home until the call for his services will be greater than ever before—for the purpose of keeping his people well, relieving them of untold suffering and financial burdens."[3]

At the very moment Shelton spoke, however, there was widespread apprehension of a physician shortage in Kentucky. From a social viewpoint, preventive medicine was considered more beneficial to a community than treatment of persons who were sick. This placed the acutely and chronically ill in a disadvantageous competition for medical care at a time when the supply of that care was declining, especially in rural areas. The country doctor of an earlier day was already a disappearing figure in 1903 when the *Bulletin of the Kentucky State Medical Association* carried the following advertisement: "DOCTOR! Do you not know you can use an OLDSMOBILE With Safety, Speed, Economy, Comfort and Pleasure." Sutcliffe and Company in Louisville was certain that physicians who realized Oldsmobile's superiority to horse vehicles would "beg, borrow or steal" the selling price of $650.[4] The automobile accelerated the general population movement from country to city, and, as rapidly developing specialization in medicine presented greater financial rewards, many doctors, and those who would become physicians, joined the general migration.

In a letter to the *Louisville Courier-Journal*, August 31, 1921, a resident of White Mills in Hardin County stated there were only one or two more doctors in the whole county than Elizabethtown had in 1900 and none were under forty years of age. High standards barred farmers' sons from medical school; those few who entered the profession from Hardin County came from wealthy families and then established their practices in Louisville. "In the course of ten or fifteen years," the writer concluded, "the people in the rural districts are going to be without physicians."[5]

Even country doctors were worried about the situation. On January 13, 1922, Dr. A. G. Lovell of Mount Vernon in Rockcastle County wrote Dr. McCormack concerning a bill for relief of the rural physician shortage about to be presented in the General Assembly. The shortage might not seem significant to city doctors, wrote Lovell, but it was a serious matter in remote districts. In his own county there were ten physicians, "all middle aged men and some beyond," who were doing all the work they could. There was no assurance the district's one premedical student would return there to practice, and even if he did the year would be 1928 according to the provisions of Kentucky's licensing law. Dr. Lovell believed the medical situation in counties comparable to Rockcastle needed "no further explanation as to what will happen in the near future unless some means of relief is provided."[6]

In perhaps the last battle of his life, Dr. McCormack rallied Kentucky's physicians to withstand a popular assault on professional prerogatives. On January 21, 1922, the state medical association's House of Delegates met in Lexington with legislators who came by special railroad car from Frankfort. Besieged by their constituents, the legislators presented the people's case chapter and verse, citing instances of counties where little or no medical care was available. Medical association leaders viewed the issue partly as a problem of physician distribution, but insisted that Kentuckians received the finest medical care. With Dr. N. P. Colwell of the AMA's Council on Medical Education present as an adviser, they stood firm on established standards for medical education. By way of compromise, the state medical practice law was amended in 1926 to provide short-term certificates for limited practice valid only in a specified county. Ostensibly the persons so certified had completed at least two or three years of medical school, but of four such practitioners in Leslie County in 1932 not one had any medical training whatsoever.

Obviously the ideal of preventive medicine was attractive when the profession was relatively weak; it became less so as it grew stronger. Specialization and the urban movement militated against community medicine under strictly professional control. And paradoxically the avenue of escape from historic professional problems by way of politics and the state ran two ways: that which was given could be taken away. By the 1920s health was a commodity to be bought in a growth economy, an idea promulgated for forty years by organized medicine. But as individuals, doctors feared a shortage of their service commodity might become a concern of the state, as indeed it already had. In 1928 the State Board of Medical Examiners reported to Governor Flem D. Sampson that there was a significant dearth of doctors in Kentucky's rural districts. Moreover, this development occurred during a relatively prosperous decade, and soon the Great Depression brought more threatening prospects. In 1932 the report of the national Committee on the Costs of Medical Care, *Medical Care for the American People*, showed that 78.5 percent of family medical expense went for treatment of illness. Such evidence and other data were construed to require reorganization of medical service under state auspices with greater emphasis on preventive medicine.

That same year, in response to a critical survey by the University of Kentucky's Department of Hygiene and Public Health, Dr. Virgil E. Simpson of the University of Louisville School of Medicine came to the profession's defense. Writing in the January 1932 issue of the *Kentucky Medical Journal*, Simpson agreed that a better distribution of doctors was desirable. There was but one 66-year-old physician for Menifee County's approximately 5,000 inhabitants and only one for Elliott County's 7,705 residents, while the ratio of physicians to population in Fayette County was 1:420. But, Simpson argued, a community deserved the kind of medical care it received. By development of its resources, both economic and social, Fayette County had made itself an attractive place for physicians and their families to settle, whereas Menifee and Elliott counties had not. The latter jurisdictions should look to themselves. Simpson also believed county governments could do much more. Each county, or at least two counties, could support a hospital offering adequate medical and surgical facilities. They could also offer scholarships to poor but talented youth whereby the state paid for premedical training at the University of Kentucky and the county assumed the cost of medical education at the University of Louisville. In accepting this aid, the student would agree to return to his or her home county and practice for a specified period.

By encouraging an exodus of doctors from Kentucky's urban

centers, Simpson thought the Depression was having a beneficial effect on the profession and on medical care. An oversupply of less successful physicians was being forced back into the country. This movement would rectify imbalances of distribution and prove the adage " 'tis an ill wind that blows no one any good."[7] He was also convinced that the suggestion of a second medical school for Kentucky was ill advised. For one thing, the taxpayers could not bear such a burden. A second school would fall below Class A standards and, in turning out poorly trained men or women, would cause better qualified doctors to leave the state. Referring to a resolution adopted by the Jefferson County Medical Society on May 4, 1931, Simpson called for public confidence in the judgment of physicians who knew best. Kentucky's medical profession had been faithful to its ideals; surely it could be trusted to lead in seeking solutions for medical problems.

The foundations of public health in the Commonwealth grew out of a concern for the high social costs of excessive morbidity and mortality which came to be recognized in the nineteenth century. Following eastern and European trends toward the use of political arithmetic and probability calculus in social administration, leading Kentucky laymen and physicians, notably Dr. William L. Sutton, secured enactment of the state's first vital statistics law in 1851. For sixty years county clerks ostensibly recorded births and deaths reported by physicians, midwives, and coroners with higher responsibility being assigned variously to the auditor of public accounts, the state registrar of births, marriages, and deaths, and finally to the State Board of Health. Many of the records required by law were never prepared; of those prepared but few were preserved, and these were arranged and stored in a manner that rendered them worthless.

Desiring financial assistance from the federal government and from private philanthropies in carrying out certain public health programs, the Kentucky General Assembly enacted the state's modern vital statistics law in 1910. By its provisions the State Board of Health was charged with legal responsibility for accurate registration of births and deaths, and it was authorized to establish a State Bureau of Vital Statistics under the direction of a registrar. This officer would divide the state into registration districts with local registrars who would then carry out the letter of the law. Regulations and instructions for reporting were made specific; those who failed to comply were liable to prosecution. Accordingly, the United States Census Bureau admitted Kentucky into the national registration area for deaths in 1911 and for births in 1918.

The 1910 law, like much of the state's significant health legislation, was drafted by Dr. Joseph N. McCormack who, together with his son, Dr. Arthur T. McCormack, provided leadership for the State Board of Health from its beginning in 1878 until World War II. Moreover, this father and son team, unmatched in the history of American state medicine, shaped the character of public health administration in Kentucky. Dr. Joseph McCormack's contribution was political, in terms of legislation and organization, at the state, regional, and national levels. As a member of the Sanitary Council of the Mississippi Valley and the National Conference of State Boards of Health, and as a powerful figure in the American Public Health Association, he worked for cooperative relations between states on health matters through organization just as he later utilized the same means to remedy internal professional problems. The passage of leadership to his son during the second decade of the twentieth century coincided with application of bacteriological methods to disease problems on a large scale. His father had established a framework for public health; Dr. Arthur T. McCormack used this framework for policy implementation and administration.

Actually death rates from infectious diseases began to decline before the bacteriological era, because of biological adaptation and newer hygienic and nutritional values that were part of a generally rising standard of living. Malaria, scarlet fever, diphtheria, and smallpox, for example, had once been serious and, on occasion, fatal diseases. They were of lesser significance in 1920, and by 1940 they had all but been eliminated by State Board of Health programs using education, vaccination, antitoxin, inoculation, isolation, drainage, and screening procedures. However, two older diseases, tuberculosis and typhoid fever, yielded less readily to natural and preventive processes, and two relatively new ones, trachoma and hookworm, threatened to arrest the state's economic and social development.

In both town and country pulmonary phthisis, or tuberculosis, was a major destroyer of health and life in 1900. Moreover since its ravages were not confined to the crowded quarters of cities or to Kentucky's poorer rural districts, Progressive Era reformers considered the disease to be of paramount social importance. Madeline McDowell Breckinridge of Lexington, granddaughter of Dr. William A. McDowell and herself a tubercular, was the leading spirit in the state's voluntary and philanthropic antituberculosis campaign until her death in 1920. Her efforts in behalf of free diagnostic clinics, school inspections, and nursing service blended into the State Board of Health's sanatoriums development program during the following decade. In 1928 Dr. Lucius E. Smith, a native of McLean County and a former medical missionary in Africa, became health officer of Breathitt County. Appalled by the extent of tuberculosis there, Smith accepted appointment as executive director of the Kentucky Tuberculosis Association in 1930, a position he held until 1951. During this service he designed treatment programs and laws and methods for prevention and saw Kentucky's mortality rate from tuberculosis fall from 94 per 100,000 of population to 33.

An early expectation that local medical societies would also serve as effective county health units proved disappointing by 1920 when the state's death rate from typhoid fever was among the highest in the nation. Though generally widespread over the Commonwealth, the disease exhibited particularly fatal concentrations in the "barren" counties near Mammoth Cave and in the mining communities of Perry and Hazard counties. Control of typhoid fever, moreover, required full-time local health organizations to carry out intensive immunization, sanitation, and educational programs. Under Dr. Arthur T. McCormack's leadership, and with the cooperation of mineowners, various philanthropies, and the Kentucky medical profession, the State Board of Health conducted a major campaign against the disease for more than a decade. Here the record shows a reduction in the total number of typhoid deaths from 657 in 1925 to 74 in 1940.

Kentucky's thirty-seven mountain counties cover an area of 13,302 square miles and in 1932 they had a population of slightly more than 800,000. The southeastern or Appalachian portion contained perhaps 200,000 persons, descended mostly from original English, Welsh, and Scotch-Irish settlers, whose customs and way of life had been shielded from public gaze until discovery of valuable mineral resources brought investment capital and industrial development around the turn of the century. A favorable tax structure and the existence of an untapped industrial labor reserve were major inducements to investment. But the prevalence of disease among the mountain people was a negative, retarding factor. By 1920 the veil of isolation covering their diseases and health practices had been lifted. These newly discovered citizens of the state were found to live in unsanitary conditions, to be superstitious believers in old midwife folklore, and to have two exotic diseases: trachoma and hookworm. These conditions called for public health measures, and from that time to the present no population group has received more attention in Kentucky's public health movement.

An infectious disease of the eye resulting in blindness if untreated, trachoma's prevalence among mountain people came to the attention of Dr. Joseph A. Stucky, a noted Lexington specialist, in 1910. Unable to act independently for want of funds, the State Board of Health appealed successfully for assistance in 1912 to the United States Public Health Service. A survey that year revealed that 500 out of 4,000 persons examined in Knott, Perry, Leslie, Breathitt, Lee, Owsley, and Clark counties were afflicted with the disease. Soon the state and federal agencies mounted programs for personal hygiene and sanitation, out-patient treatment centers, and hospitals offering surgical restoration of granule-scarred eye tissue. Between 1913 and 1925 trachoma hospitals were opened in

Hindman, Hyden, Jackson, London, and Pikeville, and in 1926 the granddaughter of Dr. Ephraim McDowell, Mrs. William McClanahan Irvine, bequeathed the family estate in Richmond for a hospital operated jointly by the United States Public Health Service, the Kentucky State Board of Health, and the Kentucky State Medical Association. Meanwhile the state and county boards of health stepped up examination clinics and other preventive activities. In 1910 about 50,000 Kentuckians were afflicted with trachoma; by 1925 the number was less than 3,000; and today the disease is no longer considered a major health problem.

Discovery of hookworm infestation in the rural South shed further light on the ills of Kentucky rural folk. A State Board of Health survey of Owsley and Larue counties in 1911 revealed the prevalence of the parasite, and soon health authorities appealed for help to the Rockefeller Sanitary Commission for the Eradication of Hookworm. During the twenty-year period 1913–1933 the Rockefeller Foundation's International Health Division supported Dr. McCormack's campaign against the intestinal parasite using treatment, the sanitary privy, and education, to the extent of $30,000. This modest investment secured the practical elimination of hookworm, like trachoma a debilitating rather than a fatal disease, as a retarding influence on economic development.

The public health spotlight on eastern Kentucky also exposed folk health practices, a high infant and maternal mortality rate, and extreme scarcity of modern medical care. Remoteness and poverty were significant factors: much of the area was inaccessible except by mule or horseback, and a 1932 study of 400 Leslie County families showed them to have a modal per capita income of $85.70. These conditions offered an unusual opportunity for a demonstration in public health; a successful program there could be duplicated anywhere. In 1925, with Dr. McCormack's encouragement, Mrs. Mary Breckinridge and other Kentucky philanthropists organized the Kentucky Committee for Mothers and Babies. Mrs. Breckinridge, a registered nurse and a London-trained midwife, had studied carefully the organization of the Queen's Nurses of

73

Great Britain, especially its program in the Scottish Highlands, and she believed that plan could be adapted to the Kentucky mountains. Its principal aim would be to reduce infant and maternal death rates by supplanting "granny" midwives with British-trained and specially licensed resident nurse-midwives.

Dr. McCormack selected Leslie County as the initial focus for the demonstration, and Mrs. Breckinridge and a few English nurses took to the hills. By 1928 the renamed and now famous Frontier Nursing Service's military uniformed nurses on horseback served families in an area of 250 square miles charging fees (payable in kind or labor) of a dollar per person per year for all nursing care and five dollars for obstetrical cases. In cooperation with the State Board of Health they also gave hookworm treatments, inoculated against typhoid and diphtheria, and chlorinated wells. During the next five years the FNS's range increased to 800 square miles, covering parts of Leslie, Perry, Clay, and Bell counties, and the scope of its activities broadened to include generalized public health nursing. Since the State Board of Health contributed but $1,800 toward the expense of this work in 1932, the main historical significance of the FNS lies in the contribution of private, voluntary philanthropy to the development of state public health programs.

Indeed, the void in preventive medicine left by the individual practitioner was filled successively by reformers and philanthropists, mostly nonmedical people, and, finally, by the public health professional. Between 1913 and 1933 Kentucky received $155,108 from the Rockefeller Foundation alone. Such gifts and grants enabled the State Board of Health to secure institutional and organizational strength through the creation of internal mechanisms. Under its auspices, for example, the University of Louisville established the School of Public Health in 1919, with Dr. Arthur McCormack as dean, to train health officers and public health nurses. The nation's and Kentucky's first full-time county health department was established in Jefferson County in 1908. Full-time development received Rockefeller support after 1920, and by 1929 there were 45 full-time departments in the state. In 1940, of Kentucky's 120 county jurisdictions, 86 had full-time health departments under the general administration of the State Board of Health. Preventive medicine as public health had become the medical specialty of the state.

7

KENTUCKY MEDICINE IN OUR TIME

THE OVERWHELMING quantities of source materials and the necessarily short-range perspectives on contemporary events make an appraisal of developments in Kentucky medicine since 1945 exceedingly difficult. It may be said with confidence, however, that during the past thirty years few issues have drawn more public, political, and professional attention in state and nation than that of adequate medical care for all citizens. A profoundly complex issue, it touches every aspect of the medical profession from education and organization to the practice of medicine itself. In this regard, one of the more dramatic developments in recent years has been the return of medical education to its Kentucky birthplace, Lexington.

Writing in the late 1870s Dr. Robert Peter, for more than twenty years professor of chemistry in the Medical Department of Transylvania University before its collapse in 1859, expressed his hope that the medical school "may yet be resuscitated when in the course of events our city again becomes an eligible site for modern medical instruction, and when special means can be obtained properly to equip and re-establish it on a basis suited to the existing times." This would entail acquisition of facilities—lacking in the past—for anatomical study and clinical teaching, to insure the fullest preparation and training of young physicians. Then, Peter prophesied, "the old

Medical College of Transylvania may revive under the wing of a people's educational institution such as Transylvania is and always was —a '*State University*.' "[1]

The political and professional issue of a second medical school for Kentucky arose during the 1920s from public apprehension of a doctor shortage and professional fears that the gains of twenty years might be lost. In 1928 Dr. John S. Chambers, a native of Calloway County and a graduate of the state university who received his M.D. degree from the University of Michigan, became both director of the University Health Service and head of the Department of Hygiene and Public Health at the University of Kentucky. For years the Lexington school had provided premedical training for students going on to the University of Louisville. But Chambers believed there was a need for more physicians and that the University of Kentucky should have a medical school of its own. In 1931 his department issued a highly critical report, *Medical Service in Kentucky*, showing a doctor shortage in rural areas that could be relieved by the establishment of a state-supported medical school. As we have seen, the report was sharply challenged by Dr. Virgil E. Simpson of the University of Louisville, a prominent medical educator and leader in organized medicine. Simpson denied the need for more doctors and expressed strong reservations about a second school.

But the issue did not die down; indeed, it became more intense as the decline in physician numbers continued. In 1940, with a population of about 2,900,000, Kentucky had 2,761 licensed practitioners. By 1950, with but a slight drop in population, the Commonwealth had 2,529 doctors, not all of whom were engaged in private practice. A special study three years later showed a total of 2,334 physicians, of whom 2,176 were classed as full-time private practitioners. Of this number all but 1,219 were specialists. Almost half the doctors were in the 40–60 age range, and of 657 practitioners past 60 there were 385 more than 70 years old.

During the early 1950s Dr. Chambers and University of Kentucky President Herman L. Donovan enlisted the support of former Governor Albert B. Chandler. No stranger to the medical care issue, a veteran of skirmishes with organized medicine, and a wily political tactician, Chandler took personal leadership of the movement for a Lexington medical school in his grass-roots bid for reelection to the governorship. In 1952 the General Assembly instructed the Legislative Research Commission to conduct "a careful and impartial study of the desirability and steps necessary for the establishment of a State-supported medical school at the University of Kentucky."[2] The commission was assisted by the Advisory Committee on Medical Education, made up of five distinguished physicians including the immediate past president of the Kentucky Medical Association, Dr. Clark Bailey of Harlan. This committee in turn had the cooperation of Dr. Chambers and the Medical School Committee of the University of Kentucky. In November 1953, the Research Commission presented an affirmative report—*Medical Education: Does Kentucky Need a State-Supported Medical School?*—to the General Assembly.

This report is important for what it reveals of the social, quantitative approach to medical care in our time. The Research Commission utilized cost-benefit analysis of distinctions it drew between medical *demand* and medical *need*. Considered to be a combination of purchasing power and social intelligence, *demand* sought supply of medical care as an open-market commodity. The commission found a substantial excess of demand over supply in the Commonwealth. *Need*, in contrast, was defined as the social totality of disease and illness occurring in the whole population irrespective of purchasing power. In the commission's view, responsible social policy should aim to minimize the economic factor in medical care, and this required that medical personnel be trained according to the *needs* of the people.

The report showed further that in 1949 the ratio of physicians to population in the United States was 1:842; in Kentucky it was 1:1,240. By 1953 the state ratio was 1:1,353. More than one-third of the citizens lived in counties where there was but one doctor for every 2,314 people; in eight counties the ratio was less than 1:5,000; and Trimble County had no doctor at all. In six urban counties where per capita incomes were highest—Jefferson, Kenton, Fayette, Campbell, Boyd, and Daviess—the physician-population ratio was most favorable. In comparison the six counties having lowest per capita incomes—Knox, Leslie, Magoffin, Martin, Owsley, and Knott —had fewest physicians. The Research Commission construed this evidence to indicate a shortage of 1,400 doctors in Kentucky and thus a need for a second medical school.

Opposition reminiscent of the unhappiness at Transylvania in 1837 came to a climax during a tumultuous public hearing on May 21, 1953. But the Research Commission was convinced that the existing situation held prospects for "little, if any improvement" and recommended the establishment of a Grade-A school of medicine in Lexington as part of the University of Kentucky.[3] Finally in 1956, after years of bitter controversy, the General Assembly made an initial appropriation for construction of the Albert B. Chandler Medical Center. That same year Dr. William R. Willard came from Syracuse University in New York to become the University of Kentucky's first vice-president for the Medical Center and dean of the College of Medicine. The first class of forty students enrolled in 1960; the hospital was completed in 1962; and in 1964 the University of Kentucky College of Medicine conferred M.D. degrees on thirty-two graduates. Dr. Peter's hopeful prophecy of a revival of the Transylvania tradition had come true.

This blending of past and present is one of the more striking features of Kentucky medicine in recent years, a situation which presents unusual opportunities for the past to speak to the present. In our time, for example, medical educators have come to appreciate anew the value of close physician-patient relationships such as Dr. Robert Pusey of Elizabethtown enjoyed during the 1870s and 1880s. Accordingly, considerable emphasis is placed on holistic medicine: treatment of the patient (rather than merely his or her disease) as a physically and spiritually integrated human being. In requiring students to gain clinical experience by assisting an established physician, recently developed family-practice programs have revived the most valuable aspect of an old tradition, apprenticeship. Clinical training is indeed an essential part of medical education. But, as Dr. Robert Peter warned in the 1850s, thorough knowledge of the basic medical sciences is equally important and should not be sacrificed.

The influence and value of medical publications in our times have advanced enormously, yet they bear a continuing relation to the past. Books and medical journals remain the major sources of information about medicine to the lay public and principal media for professional communication. Here the standard of professional and journalistic integrity raised by Dr. Edwin S. Gaillard a century ago is an inspiration to the Kentucky medical editor of today. Also today, as in the past, professional associations and societies seek to promote harmony and accord among physicians through personal contact and to provide continuing education by dissemination of scientific knowledge.

The mirage of health so earnestly pursued by early settlers is no less earnestly pursued by their descendants in our time. And if the pioneers were devoted to a tradition of home treatment and self-dosage, there is abundant evidence to show that this heritage has been faithfully preserved. Today, it is true, the Kentucky physician rarely if ever encounters dysentery, typhoid fever, diphtheria, or malaria. These afflictions have passed from the scene as a result of adaptation, a higher standard of living, and the acceptance of medical values in public health. Yet disease has by no means been eradicated: renal and heart disease, stroke, and cancer are among the doctor's major concerns in our time.

There are, to be sure, significant differences between the theory and practice of medicine a century and a half ago and that of our own day. The rational concept of disease has been greatly advanced by developments in the basic medical sciences, and the means of therapy presently available would certainly astonish a practitioner of the mid–nineteenth century. In therapeutics, however, resort to an extensive and sometimes harmful polypharmacy still persists. The therapeutic excesses of orthodox medicine during the time of Dr. John Esten Cooke serve to remind the thoughtful physician that the problem of polypharmacy has relevance in the present. On the other hand, many doctors in the 1850s found themselves in a quandary, at a time of rapid change, about medicine's responsibilities as measured against its capabilities. But they struggled with their problems with courage and resolve. As it happens, they were little different from practitioners of Kentucky medicine in our time.

Notes

Chapter 1

1. Daniel Drake, *A Systematic Treatise, Historical, Etiological, and Practical, on the Principal Diseases of the Interior Valley of North America . . .* , 2 vols. (Cincinnati, 1850; Philadelphia, 1854), 1:249.

2. Samuel Haycraft, *A History of Elizabethtown, Kentucky, and Its Surroundings* (n.p., 1960), p. 151. This account was written in 1869.

3. John Walton, ed., "John Filson's Medical Apprenticeship: 'Article of Agreement,' " *Filson Club History Quarterly* 30 (January 1956):23–24.

Chapter 2

1. Samuel D. Gross, *Autobiography of Samuel D. Gross, M.D., with Sketches of His Contemporaries*, ed. by his sons, 2 vols. (Philadelphia, 1887), 2:265.

2. Ibid., p. 350.

3. Quoted in Emmet F. Horine, *Daniel Drake (1785–1852): Pioneer Physician of the Midwest* (Philadelphia, 1961), pp. 124–32.

4. [Charles Caldwell], *Autobiography of Charles Caldwell, M.D.* (1855; reprint ed., New York, 1968), p. 354.

5. C. C. Graham to Robert Peter, February 2, 1876, typescript copy in Thomas Library, Transylvania University, Lexington.

6. Quoted in Robert Peter, *The History of the Medical Department of Transylvania University*, ed. Johanna Peter, Filson Club Publication no. 20 (Louisville, 1905), p. 54.

7. H[enry] G. Doyle, "An Inaugural Thesis on the Impropriety of Unfavourable Prognosis" (M.D. thesis, Transylvania University, 1822), pp. 1–7; John A. Ingles, "An Inaugural Dissertation on Hysteria" (M.D. thesis, Transylvania University, 1834), p. 19.

8. C. C. Graham to Robert Peter, February 2, 1876. See "Minutes of the Faculty, Transylvania University Medical Department," ms. vol., entry for Oct. 25, 1822, Thomas Library. Local "resurrection" excitement became so intense that the faculty required Dr. Dudley's students to pay an extra fee of five dollars and prohibited all matriculated students from "raising subjects for the purposes of dissection."

9. Samuel Brown to Orlando Brown, January 20, 1821; June 19, 1822, Orlando Brown Papers, The Filson Club, Louisville.

10. Peter, *History of the Medical Department of Transylvania University*, pp. 57–58.

11. Huntley Dupre, *Rafinesque in Lexington, 1819–1826* (Lexington, Ky., 1945), p. 79.

12. [Robert Peter], "To the Friends of Transylvania Medical School," *Transylvania Journal of Medicine and the Associate Sciences* 10 (January, February, March 1837):164. See also Lunsford P. Yandell, *A Narrative of the Dissolution of the Medical Faculty of Transylvania University* (Nashville, Tenn., 1837), pp. 4–31 and appendixes.

13. John Q. Anderson, ed., *Louisiana Swamp Doctor: The Writings of Henry Clay Lewis alias "Madison Tensas, M.D."* (Baton Rouge, La., 1962), p. 158.

14. Ibid., pp. 165–66, 174.

15. Daniel Drake, *Pioneer Life in Kentucky, 1785–1800*, ed. with intro. by Emmet F. Horine (New York, 1948), pp. 55, 147; Gross, *Autobiography*, 1:89–91, 2:384.

16. "Browsing in Our Archives: Three Letters by Dr. L. P. Yandell, 1838," copied for publication by Otto A. Rothbert, *Filson Club History Quarterly* 7 (July 1933):151; Samuel D. Gross, "Surgery," in Edward H. Clarke et al., *A Century of American Medicine, 1776–1876* (1876; reprint ed., Brinklow, Md., 1962), p. 132.

17. "Record of Matriculations in the Medical Department of Transylvania University," 2:n.p., Thomas Library.

18. *Annual Announcement of the Kentucky School of Medicine, Louisville, Kentucky, for the Session of 1867–68* (Louisville, 1867), pp. 8–11.

19. *Thirty-Sixth Annual Announcement of the Medical Department of the University of Louisville, Session of 1872–73* . . . (Louisville, 1872), n.p. See also *The Annual Announcement of the Louisville Medical College, Louisville, Ky., Session of 1872–73* (Louisville, [1872]), p. 16.

20. *American Medical Weekly* 4 (June 3, 1876):364–68.

21. *Kentucky University Medical Department, Announcement, 1900* (Louisville, [1900]), n.p.

22. Hampden C. Lawson, "The Early Medical Schools of Kentucky," *Bulletin of the History of Medicine* 24 (May–June 1950):174.

23. Lyman Beecher Todd, *Inaugural Address, Delivered by the President, before the Kentucky State Medical Society, at Covington, April 5, 1881* (Louisville, 1881), p. 8.

Chapter 3

1. Reuben B. Berry, "Of Dysentery" (M.D. thesis, Transylvania University, 1821), p. 9.

2. [Jefferson J. Polk], *Autobiography of Dr. J. J. Polk . . .* (Louisville, 1867), pp. 40–41.

3. Drake, *Principal Diseases of the Interior Valley*, 1:249.

4. George W. Irvin, "Vital Statistics of Marshall County, Ky.," *Western Journal of Medicine and Surgery*, 3d ser. 9 (March 1852):200.

5. Benjamin W. Dudley, "A Sketch of the Medical Topography of Lexington and Its Vicinity," typescript copy, Thomas Library; "An Inaugural Dissertation on Hysteria," p. 4. The symptoms of hysteria in women, which included signs of an independent spirit, were myriad in nineteenth-century medicine. See Ilza Veith, *Hysteria: The History of a Disease* (Chicago, Ill., 1965).

6. Dudley, "Sketch of the Medical Topography of Lexington," n.p.; Francis B. Coleman, "An Inaugural Dissertation on Cachexia Africana" (M.D. thesis, Transylvania University, 1832), pp. 2–3; [B. S. Marshall?], notebook, entry for February 26, 1846, The Filson Club; Coleman, "Cachexia," pp. 9–10.

7. Lemuel C. Porter, diary, entry for June 3, 1848, The Filson Club. See also "Doctor Lemuel C. Porter," in J. N. McCormack, ed., *Some of the Medical Pioneers of Kentucky* (Bowling Green, Ky., [1917]), pp. 171–73.

8. John Allen Parker, "An Inaugural Dissertation on Gonorrhoea" (M.D. thesis, Transylvania University, 1852), pp. 2–7. Censored (unsuccessfully) throughout, Dr. Parker's thesis has this disapproving inscription penciled upon it: "Considered by the Faculty indecent and unappropriate."

9. Hamilton County (Ohio) Medical Club, minutes, July 3, 1845, National Library of Medicine, Bethesda, Maryland.

10. Haycraft, *History of Elizabethtown*, pp. 151–52.

11. George W. Ranck, *History of Lexington, Kentucky* . . . (Cincinnati, 1872), pp. 152–53.

12. W. P. Strickland, ed., *The Backwoods Preacher: An Autobiography of Peter Cartwright* . . . (London, 1858), pp. 7–8.

13. E. H. Conner, "Chronica Medica Kentuckiensis," *Bulletin of the Jefferson County Medical Society* 19 (June 1971):31–32.

14. Anderson, ed., *Louisiana Swamp Doctor*, pp. 169–70.

15. Howard A. Kelly and W. L. Burrage, *Cyclopedia of American Medical Biography*, 2 vols. (Philadelphia, 1912), 1:199–201.

16. [John G. Jefferson], notebook, entry for January 14, 1837, Thomas Library.

17. Porter diary, 1852.

18. Algernon S. Allan, "An Inaugural Dissertation on Some of the Popular Objections to Medicine" (M.D. thesis, Transylvania University, 1846), p. 1.

19. Waller O. Bullock, "Dr. Benjamin Winslow Dudley," *Annals of Medical History*, n.s. 7 (May 1935):209; S[amuel] D. Gross, "Report of the Committee on Surgery," *Transactions of the Kentucky State Medical Society, 1852* (Louisville, 1853), p. 289.

20. Quoted in Lyman Beecher Todd, *Memoir of Doctor Orrin Derby Todd of Eminence, Kentucky* (n.p., n.d.), pp. 4–5.

21. Joseph Edwin Johnson ledgers, 4 ms. vols., The Filson Club.

22. William A. Pusey, *A Doctor of the 1870's and 80's* (Springfield, Ill., 1932), p. 86.

23. Ibid., p. 100.

24. Ibid., p. 24.

25. Ibid., p. 145.

26. Todd, *Inaugural Address*, p. 7.

27. John W. Townsend, *Three Kentucky Gentlemen of the Old Order* (Frankfort, Ky., 1946), pp. 31–34.

Chapter 4

1. *A Short Sketch of the Author's Life, and Adventures from his Youth until 1818, in the First Part. In Part the Second, A Valuable Vegetable, Medical Prescription, with a Table of Detergent and Corroborant Medicines to Suit the Treatment of the Different Certificates* (Versailles, Ky., 1825), pp. 3–4.

2. John C. Gunn, *Gunn's New Domestic Physician* . . . (Louisville, 1857), pp. 5–6.

3. Quoted in Lawson, "Early Medical Schools of Kentucky," pp. 168–69.

4. Charles Caldwell, "Thoughts on the Pathology, Prevention and Treatment of Intemperance, as a Form of Mental Derangement," *Transylvania Journal of Medicine and the Associate Sciences* 5 (July, August, September 1832):345.

5. Quoted in Emmet F. Horine, "A Forgotten Medical Editor: Edwin Samuel Gaillard (1827–1885)," *Annals of Medical History*, 3d ser. 2 (September 1940):380–81.

6. *Louisville Medical News* 2 (October 21, 1876):198; *American Medical Weekly* 5 (October 28, 1876):279–80.

7. Quoted in Horine, *Daniel Drake*, p. 197; quoted in Daniel H. Calhoun, *Professional Lives in America: Structure and Aspiration, 1750–1850* (Cambridge, Mass., 1965), p. 53.

8. Charles Caldwell, "A Valedictory Address Delivered, by Appointment, to the Lexington Medical Society, on the 10th Day of March, 1831," *Transylvania Journal of Medicine and the Associate Sciences* 5 (January, February, March 1832):31–48.

9. "Proceedings of Colledge [*sic*] of Physicians & Surgeons, Lexington, Ky.," minute book, entries for December 18, 1835, February 1, 1836, Thomas Library.

10. "Annual Address of Dr. W. L. Sutton, President of the Society," *Transactions of the Kentucky State Medical Society, 1852*, pp. 20–21.

11. Robert Peter, *A Brief Sketch of the History of Lexington, Kentucky, and of Transylvania University* (Lexington, 1854), p. 20.

12. L[ewis] S. McMurtry, "In Memoriam. Joseph Nathaniel McCormack, 1847–1922," *Kentucky Medical Journal* 21 (January 1923):3.

Chapter 5

1. "Minutes of the Forty-Eighth Annual Meeting Held at Louisville, Kentucky, April 22, 23 and 24, 1903," *Bulletin of the Kentucky State Medical Society* 1 (June 1903):3.

2. Ibid., p. 8.

3. *Acts of the General Assembly of the Commonwealth of Kentucky . . . 1904* (Louisville, 1904), Chapt. 34, pp. 100–106.

4. J. N. McCormack, "What the People Should Know about the

Doctors and What the Doctors Should Know about Themselves," *Alabama Medical Journal* 19 (December 1906):7.

5. J. N. McCormack, "The New Gospel of Health and Long Life," *Kentucky Medical Journal* 21 (January 1923):26.

6. J. R. Allen, "Rebellion in Kentucky," *Cincinnati Lancet-Clinic*, n.s. 53 (September 17, 1904):294–95.

7. "Peace on Earth, Good Will to Men," *Kentucky Medical Journal* 3 (January 1906):692; "Organization Work in Kentucky," *Kentucky Medical Journal* 3 (May 1906):813–14.

8. "Official Minutes of the House of Delegates of the Fifty-sixth Annual Session of the Kentucky State Medical Association, Held at Paducah, October 23, 24, 25 and 26, 1911," *Kentucky Medical Journal* 9 (November 1, 1911):920.

9. Ibid.

10. Abraham Flexner, *I Remember* (New York, 1940), pp. 3–36.

11. Ibid., pp. 55–56.

12. Ibid., pp. 66–75.

13. Ibid., pp. 83–111.

14. Ibid., pp. 111–21.

15. Abraham Flexner, *Medical Education in the United States and Canada* (New York, 1910), pp. 17, 146.

16. Ibid., pp. 42–43.

17. Ibid., pp. 140, 158–60, 230.

18. Ibid., pp. 178–81, 230.

19. Ibid., p. 231.

20. Quoted in David H. Banta, "Medical Education: Abraham Flexner—A Reappraisal," *Social Science and Medicine* 5 (December 1971):657.

Chapter 6

1. *Inaugural Address*, pp. 5–6.

2. Will J. Shelton, "The Progress of Preventive Medicine," *Kentucky Medical Journal* 20 (February 1922):100–101.

3. Ibid., p. 101.

4. *Bulletin of the Kentucky State Medical Association* 1 (October 1903):104.

5. Quoted in *Kentucky Medical Journal* 20 (May 1922):301.

6. Ibid., p. 300.

7. Virgil E. Simpson, "A Doctor Looks at Medical Service in Kentucky," *Kentucky Medical Journal* 30 (January 1932):9.

Chapter 7

1. Peter, *History of the Medical Department of Transylvania University*, pp. 56, 61.

2. Legislative Research Commission, *Medical Education: Does Kentucky Need a State-Supported Medical School?* Research publication no. 37 (Frankfort, 1953), p. i.

3. Ibid., pp. 20–21, 61–69.

Bibliographical Note

MATERIALS AVAILABLE to the student of Kentucky medicine are extensive and yet they are also somewhat obscure. The reason is simply that, with few exceptions, source materials for the state's medical history have not been studied. Thus very little (and even less that is valuable) has been written. In these circumstances the researcher seeking to take a synthetic approach is immediately confounded. The one comprehensive effort, compiled and written by the Medical Historical Research Project of the Work Projects Administration for the Commonwealth of Kentucky, *Medicine and Its Development in Kentucky* (Louisville, Ky., 1940), should be used with caution.

Such a statement of general conditions is qualified by the contributions of two Kentucky physician-historians. Between 1966 and 1974, under the general title "Chronica Medica Kentuckiensis," Eugene H. Conner, M.D., of Louisville, wrote about eighty carefully researched biographical sketches and short historical pieces for the *Bulletin of the Jefferson County Medical Society*. Many of them treat physicians who practiced in the Louisville area; others cover a wide range of medical subjects. The state's outstanding medical historian is the late Emmet Field Horine, M.D. (1885–1964) of Louisville. Dr. Horine published some 150 medical and historical articles during his career. He also did exhaustive editorial work on Daniel Drake's incomparable memoir, *Pioneer Life in Kentucky, 1785–1800* (New York, 1948), and thereafter published the definitive biography: *Daniel Drake, 1785–1852: Pioneer Physician of the Midwest* (Philadelphia, 1961).

At the time of his death, Dr. Horine's personal library of 20,000 volumes and other items probably embraced the finest Kentucky medical history collection in existence. By his will materials important for this essay were disposed of in the following manner: (1) the Caldwell collection went to Kornhauser Health Sciences Library, University of Louisville, which also houses the WPA collection; (2) certain Kentuckiana went to The Filson Club in Louisville; (3) the

Daniel Drake and Kentucky medical materials went to Special Collections, Margaret I. King Library, University of Kentucky; and (4) various medical works published prior to 1800 went to the Frances Carrick Thomas Library, Transylvania University. These are the principal depositories of historical materials for Kentucky medicine.

Bibliographical guides proved helpful at the beginning, and the most important were: Genevieve Miller, ed., *Bibliography of the History of Medicine of the United States and Canada, 1939–1960* (Baltimore, Md., 1964); *Bibliography of the History of Medicine 1964–1969* (Washington, D.C., 1972); J. Winston Coleman, Jr., *A Bibliography of Kentucky History* (Lexington, Ky., 1949); and Jacqueline Bull's annual compilations, "Writings on Kentucky History," published in the *Register of the Kentucky Historical Society*. Among the most useful interpretive books on Kentucky and its two principal cities are Thomas P. Abernethy, *Three Virginia Frontiers* (Baton Rouge, La., 1940); Niels H. Sonne, *Liberal Kentucky, 1780–1828* (New York, 1939); Thomas D. Clark, *Kentucky: Land of Contrast* (New York, 1968); Bernard Mayo, "Lexington, Frontier Metropolis," in Eric F. Goldman, ed., *Historiography and Urbanization: Essays in American History in Honor of W. Stull Holt* (Baltimore, Md., 1941); and Richard C. Wade, *The Urban Frontier: Pioneer Life in Early Pittsburgh, Cincinnati, Lexington, Louisville, and St. Louis* (Chicago, 1964).

The best general collection of manuscript materials important for medicine in Kentucky is held by the Filson Club, Louisville. A few of its original holdings quoted from or referred to in this essay include: Alexander M. Edmiston, letters; Henry Ellis Guerrant, papers; Edward Owings Guerrant, papers; Orlando Brown, papers; [B. S. Marshall?], notebook; Lemuel C. Porter, diary; John Bemiss, account book; Joseph Edwin Johnson, ledgers; L. P. Yandell family, papers. The manuscript holdings of the Frances Carrick Thomas Library, Transylvania University, are of a different order, but they are also extremely valuable. To mention a few items briefly: minutes of the medical faculty and of the trustees, Transylvania University; "Proceedings of Colledge [*sic*] of Physicians & Surgeons, Lexington, Ky."; lectures of Robert Peter, M.D.; "Record of Matriculations in the Medical Department of Transylvania University, 1819–1859." Also, handscript theses written by Transylvania students for the M.D. degree, 1819–1859, are bound and catalogued in Special Collections. These alone are a gold mine of research material.

Printed sources make up a large portion of primary materials, and the quantity of books and pamphlets is truly formidable. Among them are autobiographies, memoirs, published professional works by physicians, and some compilations of documents no longer easily located. Significant autobiographies include, for example, Charles Caldwell, *Autobiography of Charles Caldwell, M.D.* (New York, 1968); Samuel D. Gross, *Autobiography of Samuel D. Gross, M.D., with Sketches of His Contemporaries*, edited by his sons, 2 vols. (Philadelphia, 1887); Abraham Flexner, *I Remember* (New York, 1940); J[oseph] W. Pryor, *Doctor Pryor: An Autobiography* (Cynthiana, Ky., 1943); and [Jefferson J. Polk], *Autobiography of Dr. J. J. Polk . . .* (Louisville, Ky., 1867). Important memoirs are Daniel Drake, *Pioneer Life in Kentucky, 1785–1800*, already mentioned, and the two volumes of Robert Peter, both prepared by or with the assistance of his daughter, Miss Johanna Peter: *Transylvania University: Its Origin, Rise, Decline, and Fall* (Louisville, Ky., 1896), and *The History of the Medical Department of Transylvania University* (Louisville, Ky., 1905). An example of medical memoir pamphlet material collected by Dr. Horine is Lyman Beecher Todd, *Memoir of Doctor Orrin Derby Todd, of Eminence, Kentucky* (n.p., n.d.). A large quantity of such printed sources may be found in Special Collections, Margaret I. King Library.

Published works by physicians and others on the theory and practice of medicine constitute a large and diversified category. Indicative of breadth and scope in this area are Daniel Drake, *A Systematic Treatise, Historical, Etiological, and Practical, on the Principal Diseases of the Interior Valley of North America . . .* , 2 vols. (Cincinnati, 1850; Philadelphia, 1854); William Loftus Sutton, *A History of the Disease Usually Called Typhoid Fever, as It Appeared in Georgetown and Its Vicinity, with Some Reflections as to Its Causes and Nature* (Louisville, Ky., 1850); John Q. Anderson, ed., *Louisiana Swamp Doctor: The Writings of Henry Clay Lewis alias "Madison Tensas, M.D."* (Baton Rouge, La., 1962); and Abraham Flexner, *Medical Education in the United States and Canada* (New York, 1910). One valuable compilation of documents is J. N. McCormack, ed., *Some of the Medical Pioneers of Kentucky* (Bowling Green, Ky., [1917]).

Other important primary printed sources include annual announcements and circulars for Kentucky medical colleges and the various medical journals. The Thomas Library has a fine collection of Transylvania Medical Department circulars and it also has full runs of the *Transylvania Journal of Medicine and the Associate Sciences* and the *Transylvania Medical Journal*. The Kornhauser Health Sciences

Library in Louisville has fairly complete files of announcements and circulars for the Louisville Medical Institute (in 1846 renamed Medical Department of the University of Louisville), the Kentucky School of Medicine, the Louisville Medical College, the Hospital College of Medicine, the Louisville National Medical College, and the Kentucky University Medical Department. While it is tedious, painstaking work, careful study of the old circulars is essential to an understanding of the history of medical education in Kentucky.

The Kornhauser Library also has runs of major nineteenth-century Louisville medical journals as well as the publications (under several titles) of the state medical association. The Louisville journals include the *Western Journal of Medicine and Surgery*, the *Richmond and Louisville Medical Journal*, and the *American Practitioner*, subsequently renamed *American Practitioner and News*. The state medical association has been known as the Kentucky State Medical Society, the Kentucky State Medical Association, and the Kentucky Medical Association, its present name. Its publication has been entitled *Transactions, Bulletin of the Kentucky State Medical Society, Kentucky Medical Journal, Journal of the Kentucky State Medical Association*, and, presently, *Journal of the Kentucky Medical Association*.

A final category of printed primary sources is public documents: *Acts of the General Assembly* relating to public health and medical practice, various *Reports* of the Kentucky State Board of Health, and so forth. Two such documents having particular significance for this essay are *Guide to Public Vital Statistics Records in Kentucky* (Louisville, Ky., 1942), and Legislative Research Commission, *Medical Education: Does Kentucky Need a State-Supported Medical School?* Research Publication no. 37 (Frankfort, Ky., 1953).

A broad overview of the history of medicine and science in the United States may be gained from John Duffy, *Epidemics in Colonial America* (Baton Rouge, La., 1953); Richard H. Shryock, *Medicine in America: Historical Essays* (Baltimore, Md., 1966); Henry B. Shafer, *The American Medical Profession, 1783 to 1850* (New York, 1936); Gert H. Brieger, ed., *Medical America in the Nineteenth Century: Readings from the Literature* (Baltimore, Md., 1972); William G. Rothstein, *American Physicians in the Nineteenth Century: From Sects to Science* (Baltimore, Md., 1972); and George H. Daniels, *American Science in the Age of Jackson* (New York, 1968).

Other secondary works particularly helpful in understanding development of professional institutions are Daniel H. Calhoun, *Profes-*

sional Lives in America: Structure and Aspiration, 1750–1850 (Cambridge, Mass., 1965); Joseph F. Kett, The Formation of the American Medical Profession (New Haven, Conn., 1968); Donald E. Konold, A History of American Medical Ethics, 1847–1912 (Madison, Wis., 1962); and William F. Norwood, Medical Education in the United States before the Civil War (Philadelphia, 1944).

Secondary works having significance for Kentucky medicine include Madge E. Pickard and R. Carlyle Buley, The Midwest Pioneer: His Ills, Cures, & Doctors (New York, 1946); James T. Flexner, Doctors on Horseback (New York, 1937); William A. Pusey, A Doctor of the 1870's and 80's (Springfield, Ill., 1932); Irvin Abell, A Retrospect of Surgery in Kentucky: The Heritage of Kentucky Medicine ([Louisville, Ky.], 1926); John W. Townsend, Three Kentucky Gentlemen of the Old Order (Frankfort, Ky., 1946); Frederick Eberson, Portraits: Kentucky Pioneers in Community Health and Medicine (Louisville, Ky., 1968); August Schachner, Ephraim McDowell, "Father of Ovariotomy" and Founder of Abdominal Surgery (Philadelphia, 1921); Huntley Dupre, Rafinesque in Lexington, 1819–1826 (Lexington, Ky., 1945); Leland Arthur Brown, Early Philosophical Apparatus at Transylvania College and Relics of the Medical Department (Lexington, Ky., 1959); and Walter W. Jennings, Transylvania: Pioneer University of the West (New York, 1955).

The run of the Filson Club History Quarterly contains numerous relevant pieces, and there are a few items in the Register of the Kentucky Historical Society. For the history of the Frontier Nursing Service see Mary Breckinridge, "A Frontier Nursing Service," American Journal of Obstetrics and Gynecology 15 (June 1928):867–72. See also the agency's own publications: Quarterly Bulletin of the Kentucky Committee for Mothers and Babies; Quarterly Bulletin of the Frontier Nursing Service; and Frontier Nursing Service Quarterly Bulletin. Other journals having articles important for Kentucky medical history are Annals of Medical History; Bulletin of the History of Medicine; and Bulletin of the Medical Library Association.

Three studies originally prepared as doctoral dissertations were especially helpful in understanding personalities and in discerning attitudes and trends in Kentucky public health. These are: Mary B. Willeford, Income and Health in Remote Rural Areas: A Study of 400 Families in Leslie County, Kentucky (New York, 1932); John D. Wright, Jr., "Robert Peter and Early Science in Kentucky" (Ph.D. diss., Columbia University, 1955); and Broadus B. Jackson, "A His-

tory of Public Health Administration in Kentucky, 1920–1940"
(Ph.D. diss., Indiana University, 1963).

The purpose of this necessarily brief bibliographical note has been
to indicate the four principal depositories in the Commonwealth, and
to intimate something of their more significant contents. Most
printed materials, books, pamphlets, and journals not available in
Kentucky may be found in the Library of Congress, Washington,
D.C., and in the National Library of Medicine, Bethesda, Maryland.